Practical Hematology for BDS

Practical Hematology for BDS

Komal Marwaha MBBS MD
Reader and Incharge
Department of Physiology
Dr HSJ Institute of Dental Sciences and Hospital
Punjab University
Chandigarh, India

JAYPEE BROTHERS MEDICAL PUBLISHERS (P) LTD

New Delhi • St Louis (USA) • Panama City (Panama) • London (UK) • Ahmedabad • Bengaluru
Chennai • Hyderabad • Kochi • Kolkata Lucknow • Mumbai • Nagpur

Published by
Jitendar P Vij
Jaypee Brothers Medical Publishers (P) Ltd

Corporate Office
4838/24 Ansari Road, Daryaganj, **New Delhi** - 110002, India, Phone: +91-11-43574357, Fax: +91-11-43574314

Registered Office
B-3 EMCA House, 23/23B Ansari Road, Daryaganj, **New Delhi** - 110 002, India
Phones: +91-11-23272143, +91-11-23272703, +91-11-23282021, +91-11-23245672, Rel: +91-11-32558559
Fax: +91-11-23276490, +91-11-23245683
e-mail: jaypee@jaypeebrothers.com, Website: www.jaypeebrothers.com

Offices in India

- **Ahmedabad**, Phone: Rel: +91-79-32988717, e-mail: ahmedabad@jaypeebrothers.com
- **Bengaluru**, Phone: Rel: +91-80-32714073, e-mail: bangalore@jaypeebrothers.com
- **Chennai**, Phone: Rel: +91-44-32972089, e-mail: chennai@jaypeebrothers.com
- **Hyderabad**, Phone: Rel:+91-40-32940929, e-mail: hyderabad@jaypeebrothers.com
- **Kochi**, Phone: +91-484-2395740, e-mail: kochi@jaypeebrothers.com
- **Kolkata**, Phone: +91-33-22276415, e-mail: kolkata@jaypeebrothers.com
- **Lucknow**, Phone: +91-522-3040554, e-mail: lucknow@jaypeebrothers.com
- **Mumbai**, Phone: Rel: +91-22-32926896, e-mail: mumbai@jaypeebrothers.com
- **Nagpur**, Phone: Rel: +91-712-3245220, e-mail: nagpur@jaypeebrothers.com

Overseas Offices

- **North America Office, USA,** Ph: 001-636-6279734
  e-mail: jaypee@jaypeebrothers.com, anjulav@jaypeebrothers.com
- **Central America Office, Panama City, Panama,** Ph: 001-507-317-0160
  e-mail: cservice@jphmedical.com, Website: www.jphmedical.com
- **Europe Office, UK,** Ph: +44 (0) 2031708910, e-mail: info@jpmedpub.com

Practical Hematology for BDS

First Edition: **2010**

ISBN 978-93-80704-47-0
Typeset at JPBMP typesetting unit
Printed in India

Preface

Looking into the changed curriculum policy of DCI for BDS 1st year where physiology and biochemistry are considered as a single subject, I had felt a great need for a good workbook of practical hematology for BDS 1st year. This workbook of practical hematology is in line with the curriculum policy of DCI.

Great emphasis has been laid on the applied aspects of hematology because our aim is not to train technicians; but its aim is to make would-be dentists to learn the principles of hematology and to use them in their future clinical practice. Though students should be concerned about acquiring the necessary skill, more so in recording the results and interpreting them.

Earlier BDS 1st year students had to depend on practical physiology books or manuals which were meant for MBBS. After reading these manuals, they used to perform practical and record their results in separate practical files or note books. But the workbook *Practical Hematology for BDS* serves the purpose of textbook, manual as well as workbook. It has covered all the practical aspects of hematology.

The workbook is divided into two sections:

1. Practical section
2. Demonstrations.

The Practical section includes those practicals which are required to be included in the University practical examination. They are to be performed by the students during practical classes to acquire skills.

Demonstrations are to be shown to the students during practical classes. However, these demonstrations are not required to be included in the University examinations but questions based on this would be given in the form of charts, graphs and calculations for interpretation by the students. All the practicals are covered under the following sections.

Objectives: A set of objectives has been given at the beginning of each practical. They are intended to inform the student what they must learn from a particular exercise. The student should go through them before starting the practical and should again look at them after completing the practical, to assess whether he has acquired the necessary skill and the knowledge. The objectives covered in this book are based on what a student must know but they do not limit what he may know. Medical field being so vast, there is no end to knowledge so teachers can add on these minimum objectives.

Introduction: It covers the basic knowledge of the topic on which the practical is based.

Method: Keeping in view the fast-growing world of medical science, we want our students to remain abridged with the latest methodology used in hematology, so this section covers different methods employed for performing a particular practical. Thereafter, the detail of one particular method (required by BDS student to know) is discussed in detail. The principle of the method, all the factual knowledge and the technical data of the apparatus to be used is discussed, the whole procedure is dealt with in detail in a stepwise manner; and immediately after the procedure, sound and updated precautions to be observed are given to avoid fruitless work. After that the, way to record observation, perform calculations (if any) and express result is described.

Besides the technical details, a clear concept regarding the theoretical background of the experiment performed, its importance and uses, and clinical correlation is covered under discussion. Well-labeled diagrams and photographs of the apparatus are provided along with the text for proper understanding.

To overcome the need of using additional practical file, work space has been provided at the end of each chapter where students will record observations, perform calculations and give the results. Important viva questions are also given to help students prepare for their examination.

As far as possible, each statement included in the workbook is drawn from some well recognized source and care has been taken to cover every aspect of practical hematology BDS 1st year curriculum.

I must express my gratitude to my husband, Mr Ajay Kumar, for his endless support and understanding. I express my thanks to Jaypee Brothers Medical Publishers (P) Ltd for bringing out this workbook in excellent form. I request all the students and the teachers using this workbook to evaluate it with open mind and give their valuable suggestions.

Komal Marwaha

Contents

Plate 1

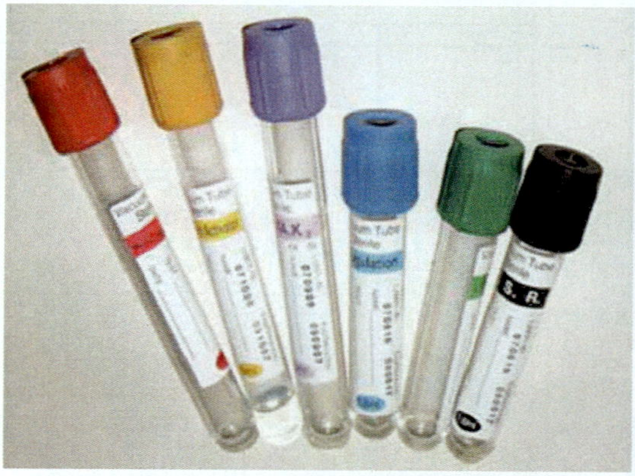

Fig. 3.1: Vaccum containers

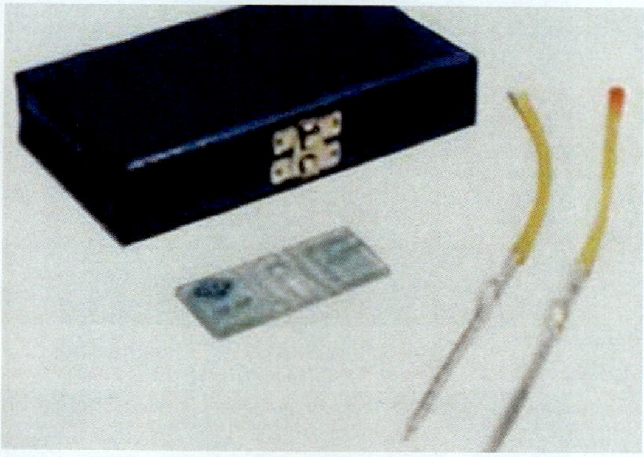

Fig. 4.1: Hemocytometer

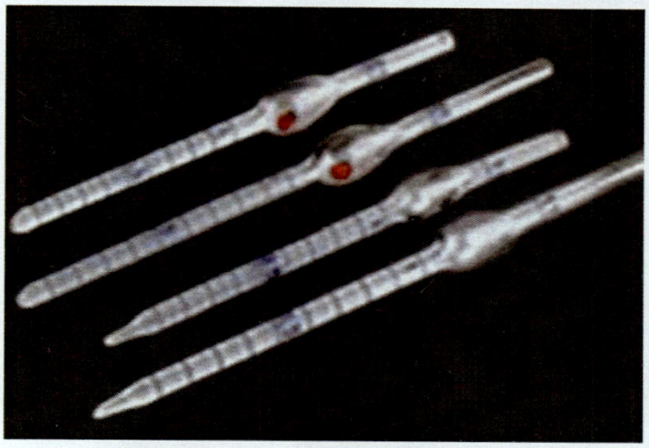

Fig. 4.2: Diluting pipettes

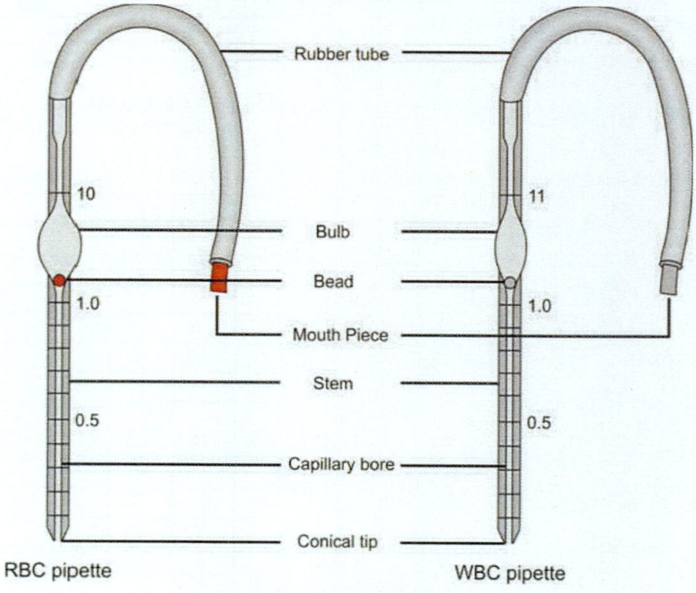

Fig. 4.3: RBC and WBC Pipettes

Plate 2

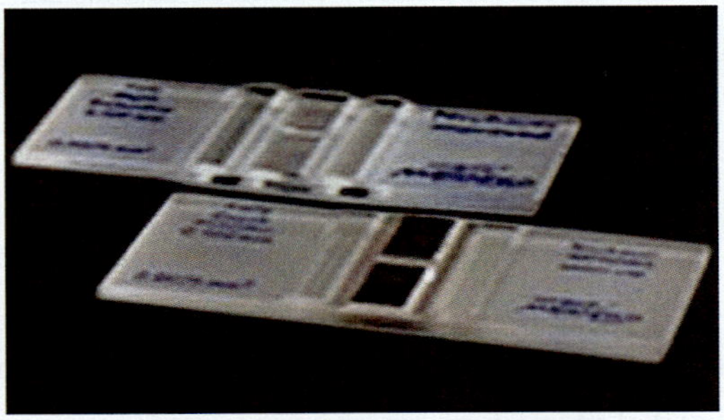

Fig. 4.4: Improved Neubauer chamber

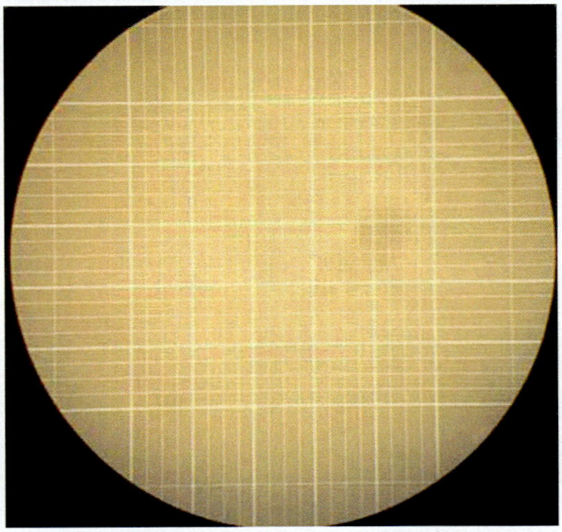

Fig. 5.1: RBC squares under 10X

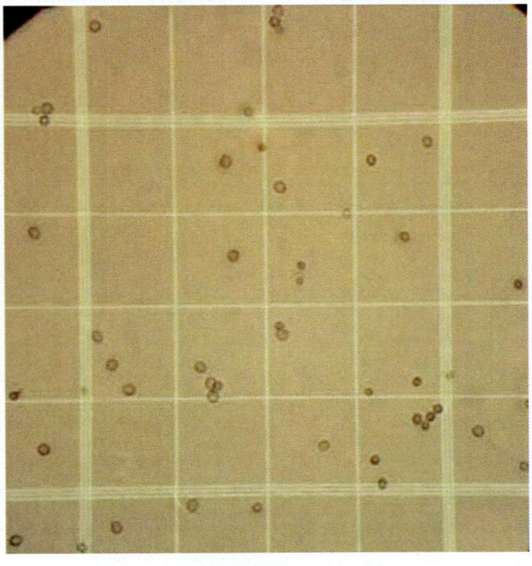

Fig. 5.2: RBCs under 40X

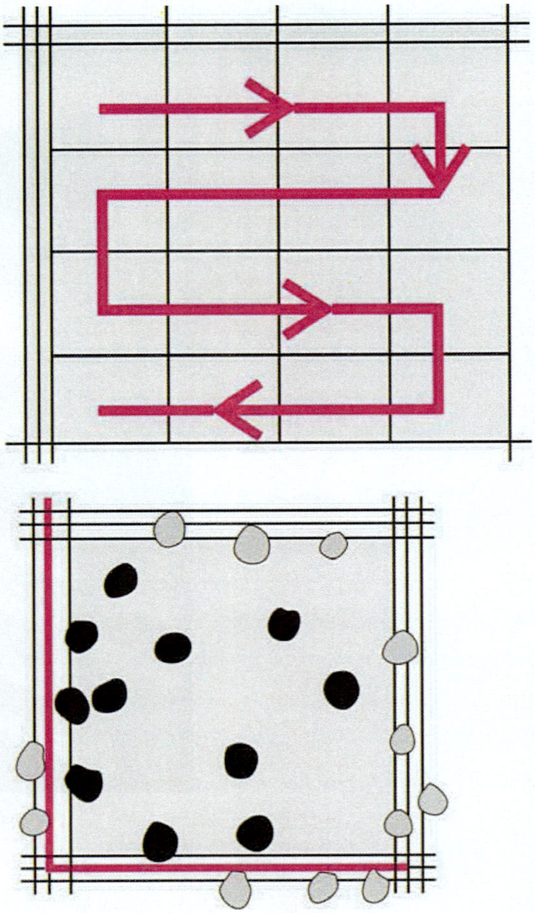

Fig. 5.4: Zig-zag way and 'L' rule of counting cells. Count the cells which are on left and bottom line

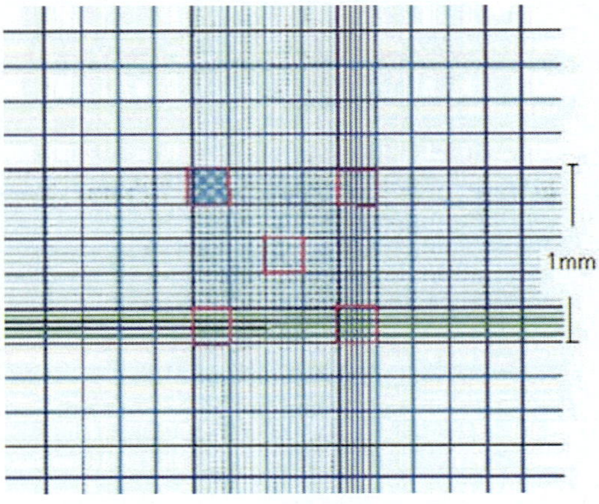

Fig. 5.5: RBC counting squares outlined in pink

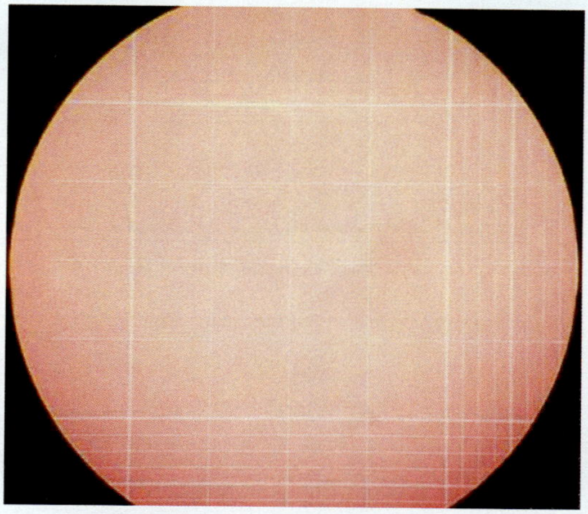

Fig. 6.1: WBC squares under microscope

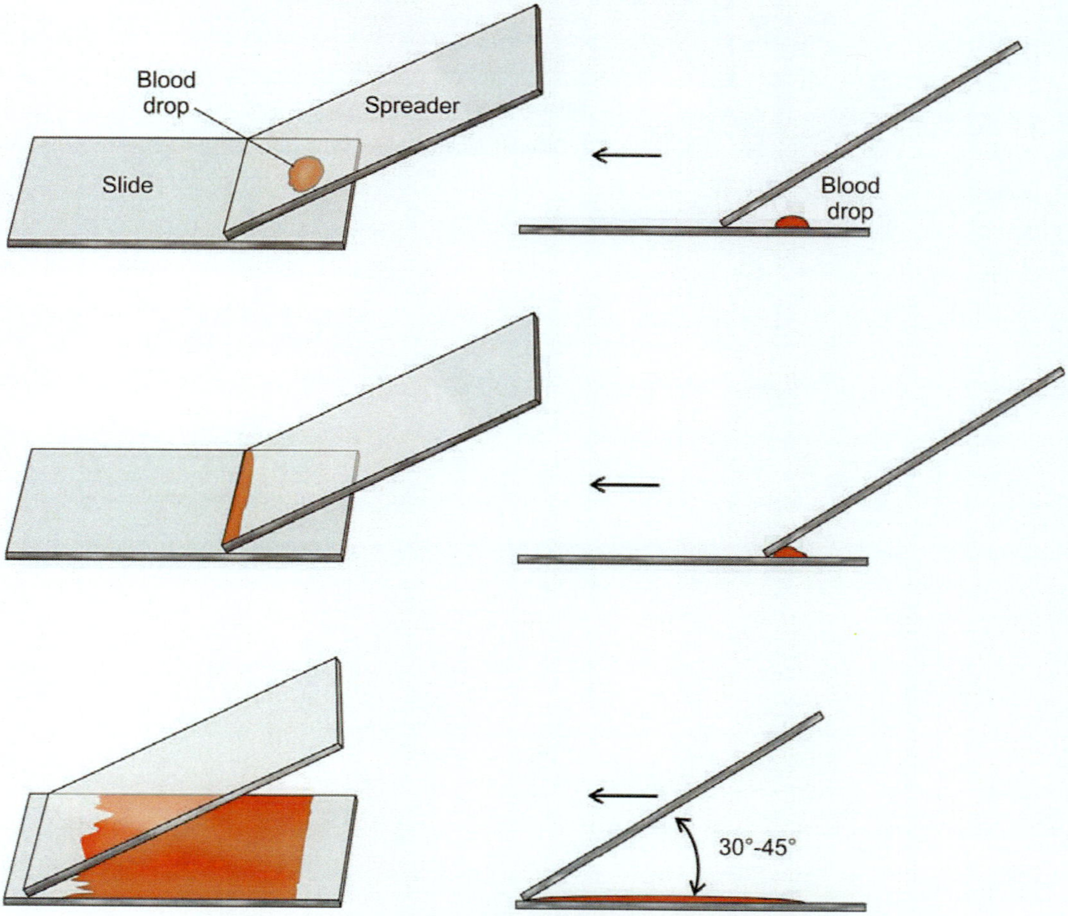

Fig. 7.1: Method of smear preparation

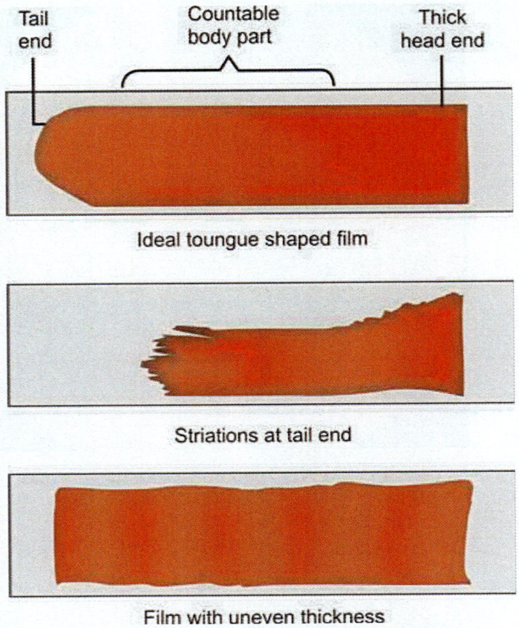

Fig. 7.2: Different types of blood films

Plate 5

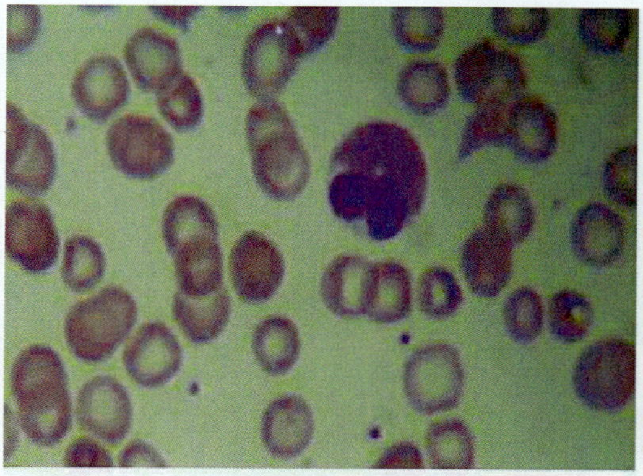

Eosinophil

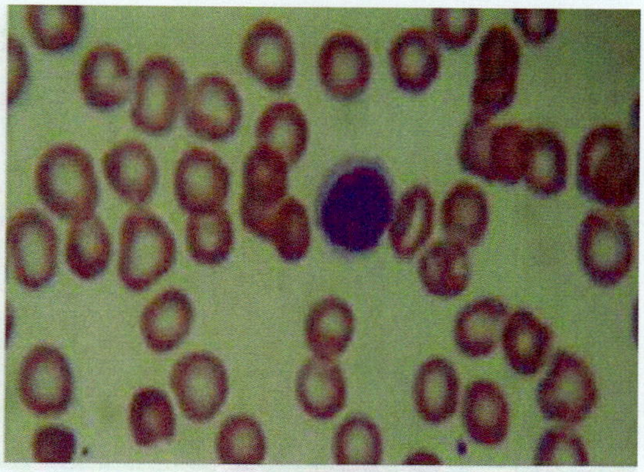

Large lymphocyte

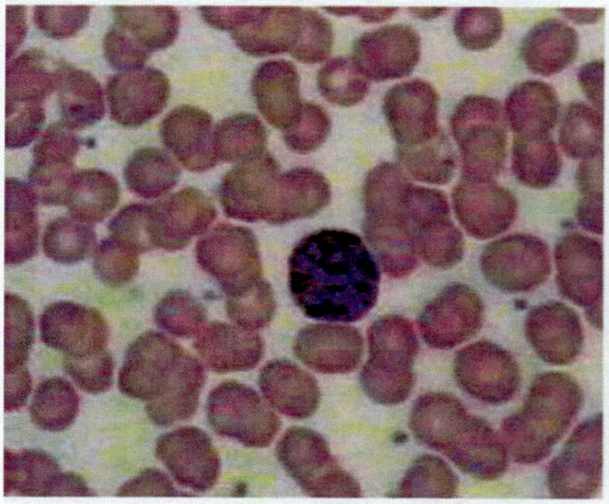

Basophil

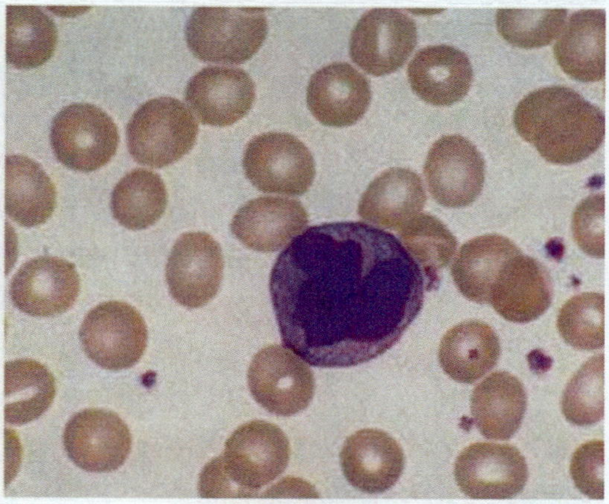

Monocyte

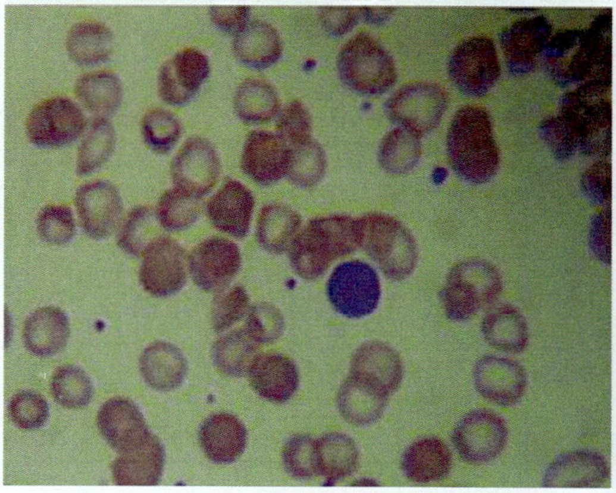

Small lymphocyte

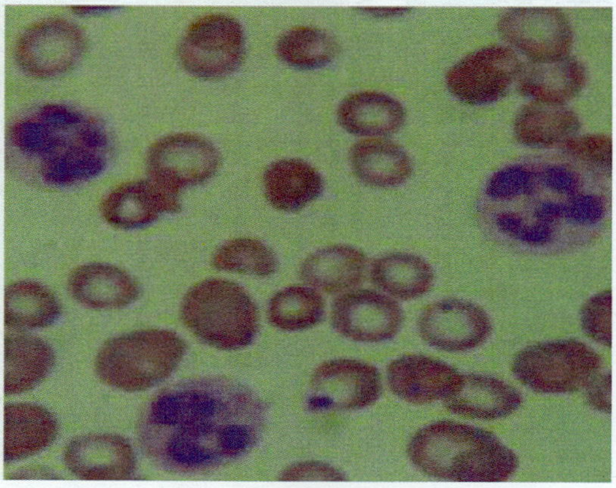

Neutrophil

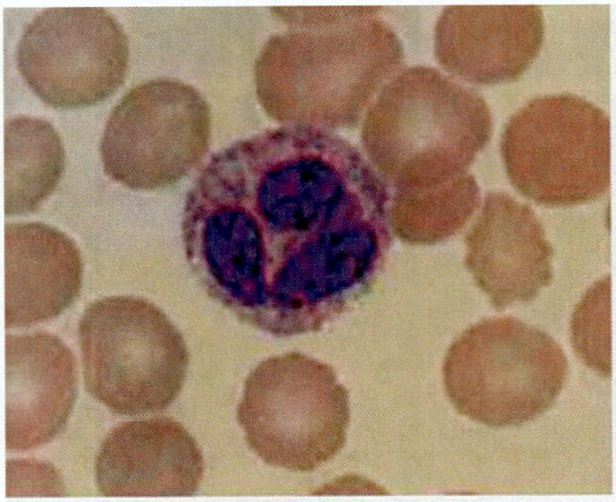

Neutrophil

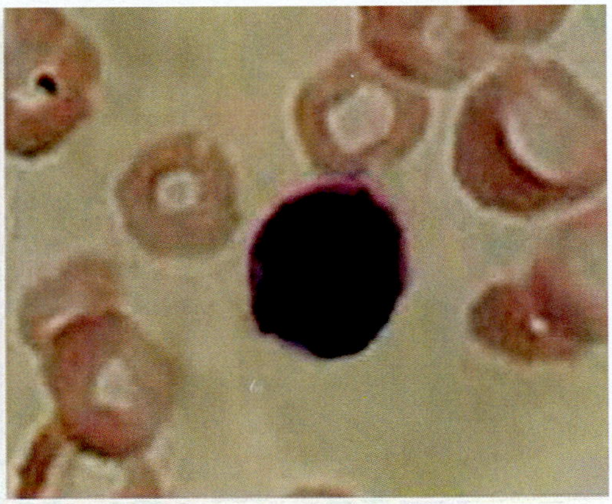

Small lymphocyte

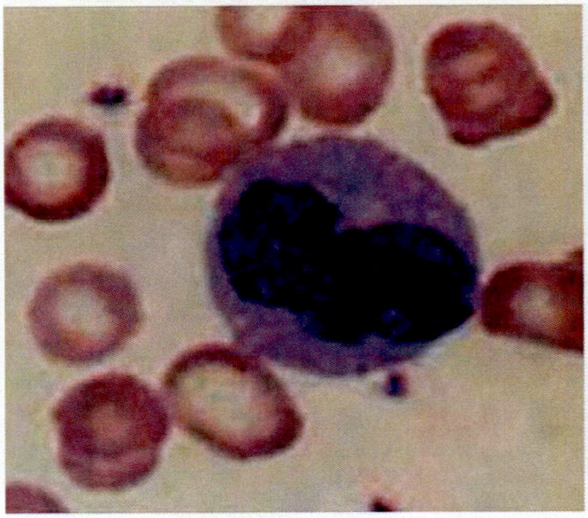

Monocyte

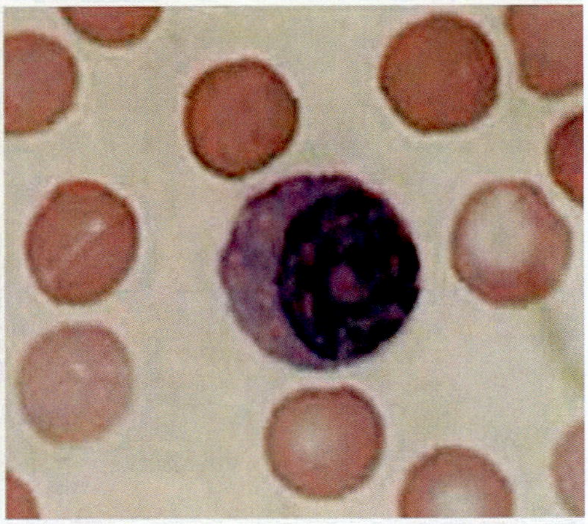

Large lymphocyte

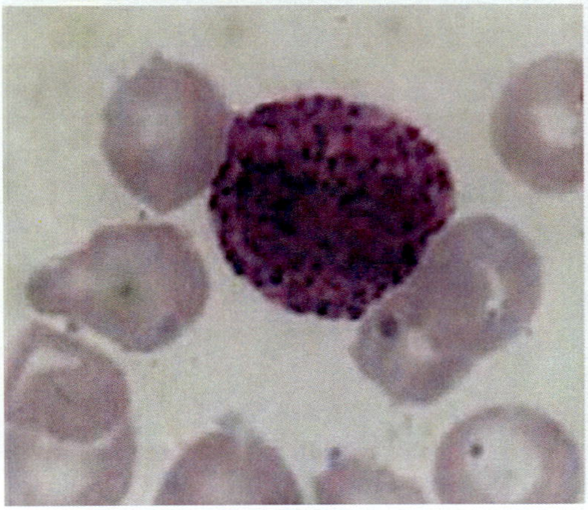

Basophil

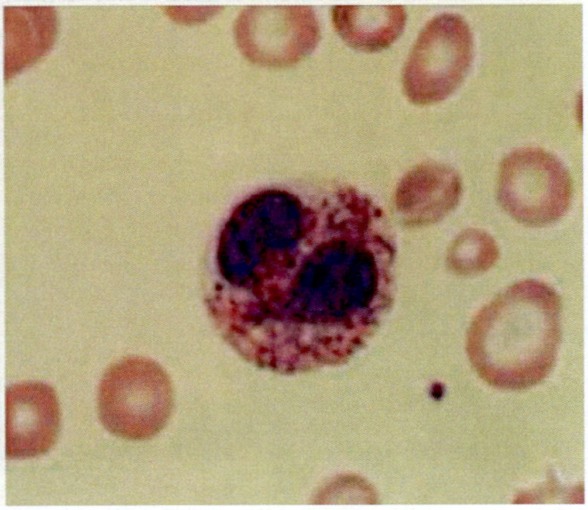

Eosinophil

Plate 7

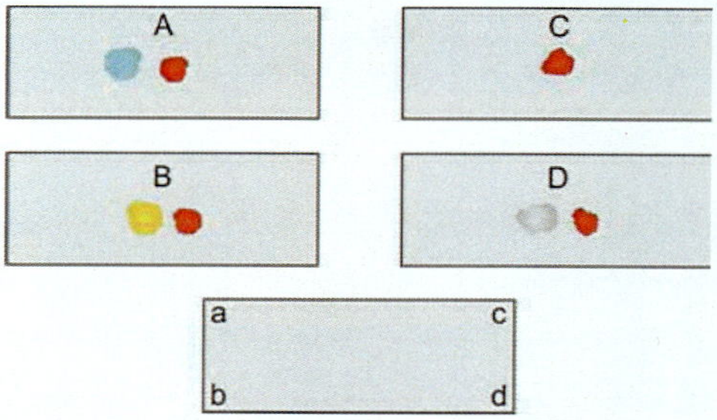

Fig. 10.1: Labelling of slides

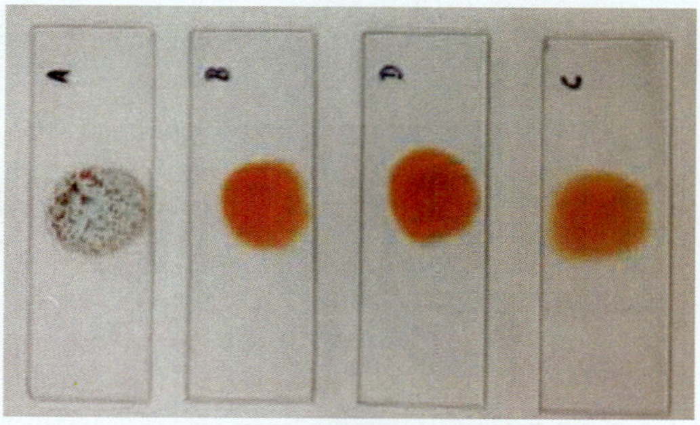

Fig. 10.3: Agglutination seen in slide A

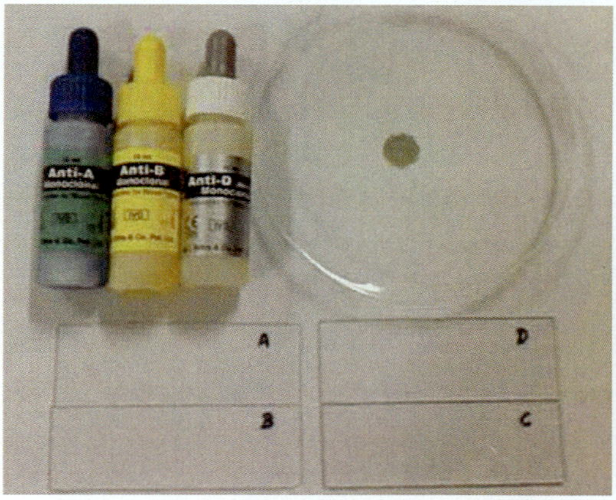

Fig. 10.2: Antiserum, watch glass and slides for blood grouping

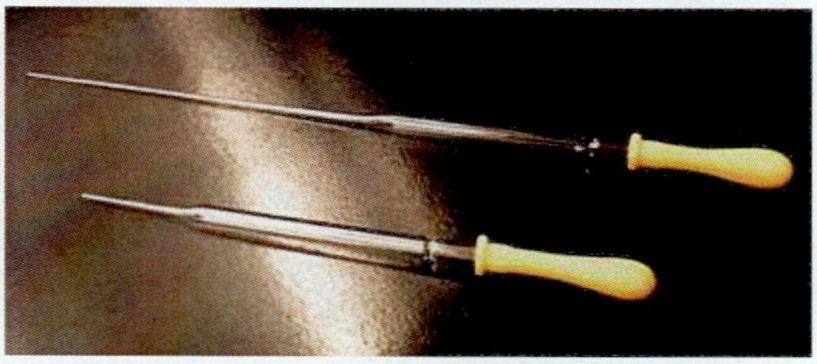

Fig. D1.2: Pasteur pipette

Practical Section 1

CHAPTER

1

Study of Compound Microscope

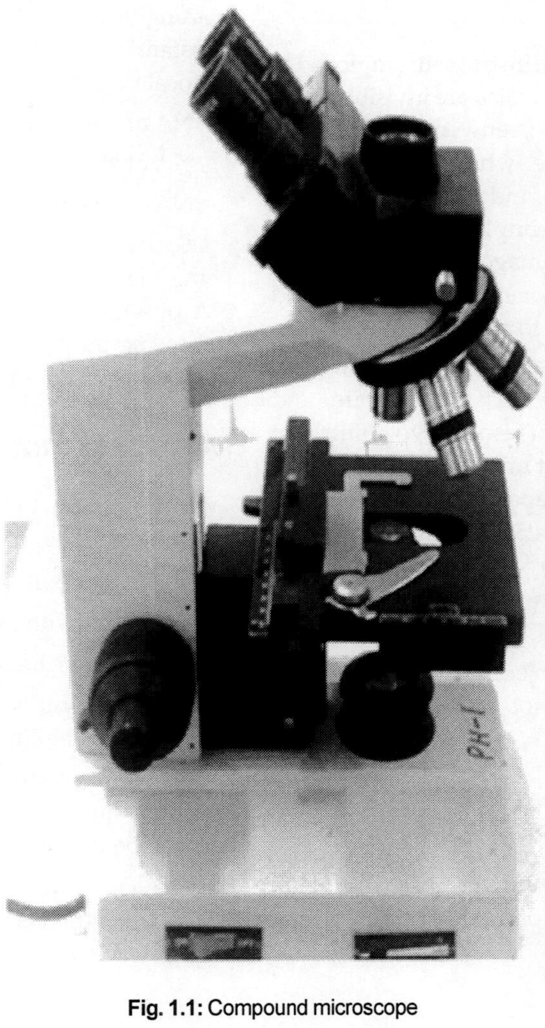

Fig. 1.1: Compound microscope

OBJECTIVE

After completing the practical student should:

- Know basics of microscopy
- Be able to identify different parts of compound microscope and state their function
- Be able to use different objective lenses with appropriate setting of condenser, iris diaphragm and lamp
- Explain the use of immersion oil for 100X **objective.**

INTRODUCTION

Microscope is a common instrument employed to see very minute objects which are invisible to the naked eye. Anton van Leeuwenhoek invented compound microscope which has two lens system—the objective and the eye piece (in contrast to one lens in simple microscope) used for forming magnified image of an object. Before learning mircoscopy, one should understand few fundamental terms to microscopy.

1. *Resolution:* It is an ability to reveal closely adjacent structural details as separate and distinct. Human eye can resolve two points that are 0.25 mm apart; light microscope can resolve points that are 0.25 µm apart. Resolution sets the limit of useful magnification of a microscope.

2. *Limit of Resolution (LR):* Resolving power of a microscope is expressed quantitatively as Limit of Resolution (LR). It is the minimum distance between two visible objects at which they are seen as separate and not in contact with one another.

$$LR = \frac{0.61 \quad W}{NA}$$

Where, W = Wavelength of light rays

NA = Numerical aperture of objective lens in use.

3. *Numerical Aperture (NA):* NA of a lens is an index of its resolving power. Greater the numerical aperture, greater is the resolving power. As NA increases, the resolution distance (distance between two objects at which they can be seen as separate and distinct) decreases.

Numerical Aperture can also be described as an index of light gathering power of a lens, i.e. amount of light entering the objective. NA of the lens is the ratio of diameter of the lens to its focal length. NA can be increased or decreased by increasing or decreasing the amount of light passing through a lens. Any particular lens has constant NA, which depends on its radius and its focal length.

NA of Low power objective lens = 0.30

NA of High power objective lens = 0.65

NA of oil immersion objective lens = 1.30

Focal Length: It is the distance from the object being viewed to the objective lens. Change in NA of lens can be achieved by decreasing or increasing the FL as radius of the lens fitted in microscope cannot be changed.

PARTS OF MICROSCOPE

Two types of Compound Microscope are commonly used.

1. Monocular (with one eye piece)
2. Binocular (with two eye pieces).

Both types have these parts.

1. *Base:* Usually it is horseshoe shaped. It gives support and stability to the microscope.

2. *Handle:* It supports the magnifying system and the adjusting system of the microscope. It can also be used for carrying the microscope.

3. *Body Tube:* It is a cylindrical tube through which light travels. Its length determines the mechanical length (distance between upper part

of objective lens and eye piece) of microscope. Increase in tube length increases the magnification but this may result in loss of clarity of image. The tube length is therefore fixed which is normally 160-170 mm. Tube consists of 2 parts:

- *Outer tube:* It bears nosepiece at its lower end to which three objective lenses are fitted.
- *Inner tube:* It carries eyepiece at its upper end having magnification of 5X or 10X. Inner tube can be slid inside the outer tube to adjust the mechanical length.

4. *Stage:* It has two parts

- *A fixed stage:* It is a horizontal platform on which object being observed is placed. There is an aperture in the centre through which a converging cone of light passes.
- *Mechanical Stage:* It is fitted on fixed stage. It has a spring-mounted clip to hold the slide or counting chamber in position. There are screws present for moving it to and fro and side ways.

5. *Sub stage:* It lies below the stage; it has a condenser and a diaphragm.

6. *Condenser:* It is a system of lenses, which focuses light (condenses parallel rays of light into a beam of light) from a light source on the object. It also helps in resolving the image. It is mounted below the stage of the microscope with a rack and pinion mechanism. Raising or lowering the condenser can vary the intensity of illumination of object. It must be correctly positioned to focus the light properly on the object being viewed. Being a lens, it has a fixed numerical aperture. For better resolution numerical aperture of condenser should be equal to or slightly less than the numerical aperture of the objective lens being used. So, the position of condenser must always be adjusted with each objective lens being used, to get maximum focus of light and accurate resolving power of microscope.

Table 1.1: Types of objectives and position of condenser

Types of objective used	*Position of condenser*
Low power (10x)	Lowest level
High power (40x)	Raised optimally to mid level
Oil immersion objective (100x)	Raised fully to highest level

7. *Iris diaphragm:* It is located at the bottom of condenser. It has an aperture, which can be opened or closed for adjusting amount of light that passes to the field under observation. Regulating the light by adjusting diaphragm (by reducing field size with the help of iris diaphragm) affects the NA of condenser

8. *Nosepiece:* Fixed nosepiece is attached to the lower end of the tube and revolving nosepiece is mounted under it. The revolving nosepiece carries the objective lenses of different magnifying power.

9. *Lenses:* The total magnification produced by compound microscope is the product of magnification caused by objective lens and eyepiece.

- *Eyepiece:* It is fitted into the top of the body tube. In case of binocular microscope there are two eyepieces. One of the eyepieces (the pointer eyepiece) has a pin mounted in it, which is used for indicating any cell in the field of view. Each eyepiece has 2 lenses one mounted at the top and other at the bottom.
- *Objective Lenses:* There are three spring-loaded objective lenses fitted with a revolving nosepiece.
  - Low Power Objective 10x, magnifies image 10 times
  - High Power Objective 40x, magnifies image 40 times
  - Oil Immersion objective 100x, magnifies image 100 times

Low Power objective lens 10X

- Magnifies image 10 times
- Used for initial focusing
- NA (0.3) is less than that of condenser
- To achieve maximum focus NA should be matched to that of condenser so the condenser should be fully lowered and the light has to be reduced by keeping the iris diaphragm slightly open
- Total magnification achieved is 100 times (with 10x eye piece).

High Power objective lens 40X

- Magnifies image 40 times
- Used for broad view of blood films and RBC counting etc
- NA (0.65) is almost close to that of condenser
- Condenser should be slightly raised and iris diaphragm partially opened to achieve maximum focus
- Total magnification achieved is 400 times (with 10x eyepiece).

Oil immersion lens 100X

- Magnifies image 100 times
- Oil immersion objective is used for detailed morphological examination of blood films and to obtain greater details of an object
- NA of oil immersion lens (1.30) is more than that of condenser
- Condenser should be placed at highest position and iris diaphragm should be fully opened
- Total magnification is 1000 times (with 10X eye piece)
- Its use requires special oil called immersion oil, which is placed between objective lens and slide. Commonly used immersion oils are cedarwood oil with Refractive Index (RI) of 1.51, and glycerin RI = 1.30. Liquid paraffin can also be used. Lens has to be immersed in oil during use. If we don't immerse the objective lens in immersion oil, there will be air between the slide and oil, the light will pass from glass slide (a denser medium) into thin layer of air between slide and oil immersion objective (a rarer medium, RI = 1.0). It will get refracted away from normal. So when light rays emerge from the slide, many of them will be refracted away from small aperture of oil immersion objective and very few will enter it, which will result in a faint image. If this air could be removed by a transparent liquid medium having same RI as that of glass slide and objective lens there would be no such refraction and enough light would enter the objective thus giving a clear and bright image. This purpose is achieved by using cedarwood oil, which has same refractive index (RI) as that of glass, i.e. 1.51.

Par Focal System

Objective lenses are so constructed that when one lens is in focus, other lenses are also more or less in focus. Thus switching over from one lens to another requires only a turn or two of fine adjustment screw to bring the objective into sharp focus. This arrangement of lenses is called Par focal system.

10. *Coarse adjustment screws:* They are mounted on the sides of handle by double side micrometer mechanism. On rotating one, other screw is also rotated. They can be used to raise or lower the stage of microscope quickly to obtain an approximate focus.

11. *Fine adjustment screws:* Two screws are mounted close to coarse adjustment screws by double side micrometer mechanism. They are used for exact sharp focusing.

12. *Illuminating system:* Compound microscope is a bright field light microscope where viewed objects look dark or colored contrasted against a lighted background. It uses white light which can be either external or internal.

- *Internal source:* Electrical lamp is attached at the base of microscope directly under the stage.
- *External source:* It can be in the form of electric lamp or direct sunlight. Microscopes using external source of light have mirror attached at the base to reflect light into condenser. Mirror has two surfaces; plane used for oil immersion objective and distant light source (direct sunlight) and concave for close source of light, e.g. electrical lamp and high power objective.

We require different degrees of illumination when using a microscope. The clarity of image depends upon optimal amount of light available. Raising or lowering the condenser and opening or closing the diaphragm can also alter illumination. A proper combination of two has to be selected under different conditions. In general less illumination is required for viewing a clear, unstained object, and more illumination is required for viewing a stained preparation

Method of Using Microscope

1. Place the slide on the fixed stage with object to be viewed over the central aperture.
2. Start with low power objective. By rotating nosepiece bring it into position. It will come in place with a click sound.
3. Make appropriate adjustments of condenser and diaphragm.
4. Use coarse adjustment screw to bring the object into focus and fine adjustment screw for sharp focus.
5. For examining the whole slide use the screw attached to mechanical stage for moving the slide sideways and to and fro.
6. After seeing under low power objective lens, proceed to examine under high power by making appropriate adjustments of objective, condenser and iris diaphragm. Use fine adjustment for sharp focusing.
7. For oil immersion objective, swing away the high power and put a drop of cedar wood oil over the slide.
8. Bring oil immersion objective to position.
9. Raise condenser to highest level and fully open the iris diaphragm.
10. By using coarse adjustment screw and looking from the side carefully lower the objective till it just touches the oil drop.
11. Lower the objective further down to the slide.
12. Increase the gap between slide and objective to bring object into focus.
13. Use fine adjustment screw for final focusing.
14. Rack the microscope as the cells and their constituents are three dimensional structures and lie at different levels. It is important to continuously "rack" the microscope (keep rotating fine adjustment screw) once the specimen or object being viewed has been focused under any magnification. By racking they will come into and go out of focus alternatively. In this way no cell will be missed.

Precautions

1. Eyepiece and objective should never be cleaned with paper tissue or gauze. They should be cleaned with lens paper only.
2. Never touch the lenses with fingers.
3. Remove oil from oil immersion objective immediately after use by wiping it with a clean lens paper.
4. Use little of xylene to remove hardened oil if present.

5. Use of excess of xylene or benzol should be avoided. It loosens the cement material in which lenses are fitted.
6. While changing position of objective it should always click into position.
7. Always look from side while bringing down the oil immersion objective. Never lower the tube while looking through eyepiece.
8. Make proper adjustments of condenser and diaphragm for each objective for proper illumination.
9. Once a slide has been focused, use only fine adjustment for racking the microscope.
10. Never tilt microscope when counting cells in counting chamber, or when using immersion oil.
11. Carry microscope by holding its handle with one hand and keeping other hand under the base.
12. After use always cover the microscope.

DISCUSSION

Sources of Error

Inability to Focus an Object

It can occur:

1. If the object being viewed is not placed within the focal distance of the objective.
2. If the slide carrying the object has been placed upside down on the microscope stage.
3. If thick cover slip is placed over the object.
4. If the object is covered with layer of dried oil or dirt.

Unclear Image Under Oil Immersion when it is Clear under Other Objectives can Occur

1. If sticky/old immersion oil is used which will decrease visibility.
2. If dried oil (lens left unclean from the previous use) is adhered to oil immmersion objective.
3. If there is air bubble in immersion placed over the slide. It will produce dark shadow in the field of view.

Poor Illumination

Most commonly it is due to faulty combination of adjustment of the condenser, iris diaphragm, lamp or the type of mirror being used. Normally the combination should be:

Objective	Condenser Position	Diaphragm	Mirror
Low power (10x)	Lowest level	Slightly open	Concave
High power (40x)	Raised optimally to mid level	A little more open	Concave
Oil immersion objective (100x)	Raised fully to highest level	Fully opened	Plane

An Oval Field of View

This can occur if the objective lens being used is not properly clicked into position.

A Smudge in the Field can be due to

1. Dirt on slide
2. Dirty objective, if the smudge moves with the field.

DIFFERENT TYPES OF MICROSCOPES

Based upon the illuminating system there are different types of microscopes.

- *Bright field or Light Microscope:* It uses white light either external or internal.
- *Dark field microscope:* It is used for examination of unstained microorganisms. Condenser is darkened in the center and

oblique light rays pass through the periphery illuminating the microorganisms

- *Fluorescent microscope:* Object being viewed is attached to a fluorescent dye which glows when exposed to the light.
- *Electron microscope:* It is used for the study of ultra structural details of the cells. By using electron beam of light the resolving power of the microscope is increased to 50,000 to 100,000 times and very small structure can be visualised.
- *Ultra microscope:* Ultraviolet light is used which because of low wavelength gives higher magnification and the image can be viewed on the fluorescent screen.

WORK SPACE

Q1. According to the objective in the use what adjustments should be made in the position of condenser and diaphragm?

Objective lens	*Position of condenser*	*Position of diapragm*

Q2. Give different conditions in which plane and concave mirrors are used.

Type of mirror	*Condition*
Plane	
Concave	

Q3. What is the reason for changing in the position of the condenser with the change in objective lens used?

Q4. What precautions are taken when using oil immersion objective?

VIVA QUESTIONS

Q1. What is numerical aperture? Give its significance.

Q2. Define resolution.

Q3. What is Par focal system?

Q4. What is the principle of using immersion oil?

Q5. Name the fluids which can be used for working under Oil immersion lens.

CHAPTER

2

Collection of Blood Sample

OBJECTIVE

After completing the practical student should:
- Know different methods and different sites of blood sample collection
- Know the importance of each method
- Be able to collect capillary blood from finger prick
- Know about all aseptic precautions needed to be taken for sample collection.

INTRODUCTION

For obtaining blood sample skin has to be punctured and this may pose a danger to infection. It is very important to create asepsis before sample collection. Consider all samples as potential source of infection and ensure that blood should not come in contact with your body.

For routine hematological examination commonly taken blood samples are:
- Capillary blood sample
- Venous blood sample.

CAPILLARY BLOOD SAMPLE

Capillary blood is taken when the quantity of blood required is small. Tests performed by using capillary blood are:
- Determination of blood group , BT and CT
- Hemoglobin estimation
- Blood counts: erythrocytes, leukocytes and differential leukocyte count
- Platelet count
- Reticulocyte count
- Smear prepration for basophilic aggregations
- Thick smears for malarial parasites.

Source

Blood sample in adults is collected from the fingertip or the ear lobe. In infants heel is preferred.

Apparatus

1. Disposable sterile lancet.
2. Methylated spirit.
3. Dry gauze.
4. Disposable gloves.
5. Slides or graduated pipettes.

Procedure

1. Allow the subject to sit comfortably.
2. Wear disposable gloves.
3. Select the finger for puncture. It is preferable to puncture any of the middle three fingers.
4. Rub the distal digit of finger to be pricked.
5. Clean the digit with spirit swab. Allow it to get dry.
6. Hold the finger firmly and prick its distal digit by quick single 3-5 mm deep stab.
7. Wipe the first drop of blood with dry gauze.

8. Do not squeeze the pricked finger. Let the second drop form slowly and spontaneously.
9. Rapidly collect the blood sample either on the slide or in the pipette as the case may be.
10. Press fresh dry gauze on the punctured site till the bleeding stops.

Precautions

1. Take all aseptic precautions.
2. All instruments to be used for sample collection – lancet, needle, syringe, gauze, etc. should be sterilized.
3. Site of puncture should always be cleaned with methylated spirit. Once the site has been cleaned it should not be touched again.
4. Choose any of the middle three fingers because palmar fascia of middle three fingers is limited to hand only(whereas that of thumb and little finger is continuous with that of arm), if infection occurs following puncture it will be limited to the hand only.
5. Finger chosen should be free from any skin disease, injury, inflammation, etc.
6. Rub the finger before pricking to improve circulation (especially if the fingertip is cold).
7. Finger tip should be punctured only after it is completely dry because:
   - Sterilization by alcohol is effective only after it has dried up
   - Blood cells will get hemolyzed if they come in contact with spirit
   - On wet fingertip blood will spread sideways along with spirit and spherical drop which is important for pipetting will not form.
8. Prick the fingertip away from nail bed.
9. Never squeeze the fingertip after it has been pricked because squeezing will exude tissue fluid which dilutes the blood sample.
10. Always wipe the first drop of blood with dry gauze as:
    - It is diluted with tissue fluid and interferes with laboratory findings
    - It may also contain epithelial cells which will appear as artefacts on microscopic examination.

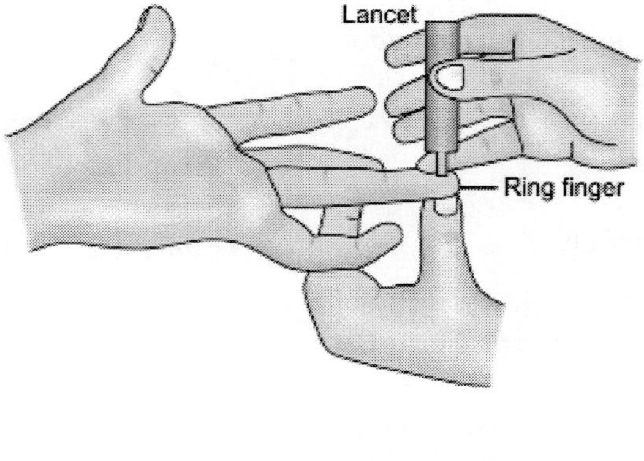

Fig. 2.1: Collection of capillary blood by finger puncture

Ear Lobe Puncture

Blood flow in ear lobe is slow and concentration of cells here is greater so it is preferred for forming blood films for DLC and to study morphology of cells but not for Hb estimation, TLC, RBC count (can give false high results). Blood taken by pricking skin comes from capillaries, very small arterioles and venules.

Procedure

1. Warm the puncture site by rubbing between fingers.
2. Clean with spirit swab and let it dry.
3. Make a quick puncture of about 2 mm depth with the help of sterile lancet.
4. Wipe the first drop and collect sample when the blood starts flowing spontaneously.

Precautions

1. Take all the usual precautions required for collecting capillary blood sample.

Heel Puncture

This is preferred site in infants because blood supply is limited in fingertips and removing blood by venipuncture would deplete too much of their blood.

Procedure

1. Place neonate on stomach if possible and place his/her limb lower than the level of the heart to increase blood flow to the foot.
2. Warm the heel for 3 minutes prior to puncture by wrapping a moist warm wash cloth up to 41°C around the heel (Moist heat helps to increase blood flow to the area) or vigorously scrub the entire foot bottom to promote circulation.
3. Clean the heel with spirit. Let it dry.
4. Hold the heel firming and puncture (2 mm deep) at a 45-60° angle on the most medial or most lateral portion of the plantar surface.
5. Wipe away the first drop of blood. Let the second drop form spontaneously.
6. Collect sample and apply pressure to stop bleeding.

Precautions

1. The blood specimen must be collected immediately after the 3 minute warming, because the wash cloth will rapidly cool the heel as it cools and this will actually slow the blood flow.
2. The antiseptic should remain in contact with the skin for at least 1 minute and should be rubbed off with a dry, sterile swab. If the site is not dried well, the antiseptic can mix with the specimen and the blood will not "bead up" well at the puncture site. Rather, the blood will spread over the moist area, making it difficult to collect.
3. The depth of an infants heel skin puncture should not exceed 2.4 mm to avoid hitting a bone. Beside protecting the calcaneum, this depth is adequate to reach the capillary beds.
4. Don't use any surgical blade for skin puncture because of the danger of a deep puncture, infection, and damage to the infants calcaneum.

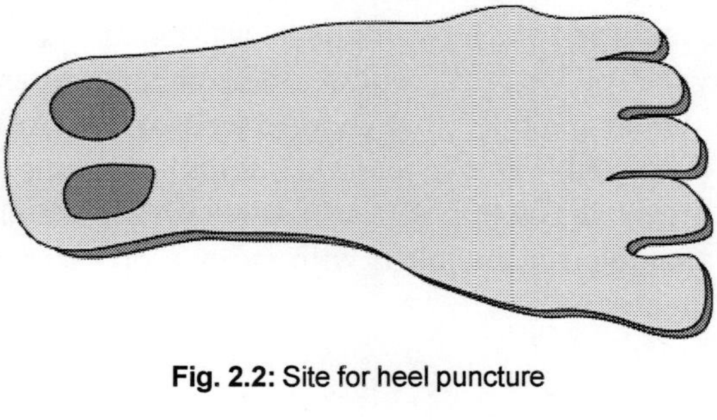

Fig. 2.2: Site for heel puncture

5. Lancets with permanently retractable blade or needle which provide a puncture of 2 mm deep and 2.0-2.5 mm in length should be preferred. These lancets are designed with guards to prevent deep punctures thus minimizes the possibility of injury.
6. Don't puncture central plantar surface and posterior curvature of the foot as this may injure underlying bones. In short heel, puncture should be on the most medial or lateral portions of the plantar surface of the heel; no deeper than 2.4 mm; not on the posterior curvature of the heel; and not through previous puncture sites that may be infected.

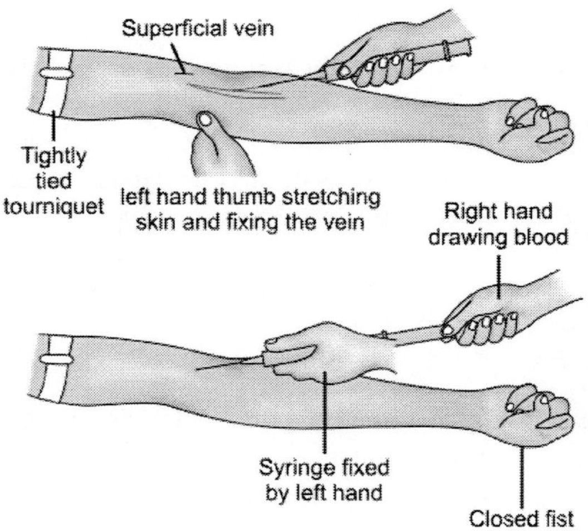

Fig. 2.3: Collection of venous blood sample

VENOUS BLOOD SAMPLE

Venous sample is taken when larger amount of blood is required for various biochemical or hematological investigations like:
- For determination of PCV
- For determination of ESR
- Determination of osmotic fragility of RBC

Source

Blood sample can be obtained by performing venipuncture of veins of:
1. Forearm
2. Wrist
3. Ankle

Venipuncture should always be done by a medically qualified person. Forearm is the most preferred site for venipuncture (Median cubital vein of forearm) because veins of forearm are larger and fuller than those of wrist and ankle. If no suitable vein in forearm is found select one of the veins on opposite arm, leg or wrist. Venous sample can be taken with syringe or vacuum tubes.

Collection of Venous Blood Sample Using a Disposable Syringe

Apparatus

1. Disposable syringe with a needle
2. Methylated spirit
3. Sterile gauze
4. Collection vial containing anticoagulant
5. Disposable gloves
6. Tourniquet

Procedure

1. Explain the procedure to the subject and take his/her consent.
2. Make him sit on the chair with his arm (palm upward) resting over armrest/table or ask him to lie down on a couch.
3. Select suitable vein in the forearm.
4. Ask the subject to clench his fist and apply a tourniquet just above the elbow.
5. Clean the area over the vein with spirit swab and allow it to dry.

6. Place the thumb of left hand at lower end of cleaned area and stretch down the skin over the vein to fix it.
7. Select the puncture site. Insert needle with the bevel upward at 30° or less and push it gently along the length of vein. On entering vein there's sudden loss of resistance.
8. Loosen the tourniquet once the needle has been inserted into the vein and blood starts appearing in the barrel.
9. Pull back the piston to withdraw required amount of blood.
10. Remove tourniquet, while the needle is still in vein and tell the patient to open his fist.
11. Gently remove needle from the patient's vein.
12. Press puncture site with dry gauze.
13. Tell the subject to flex arm for some time.
14. Remove needle from syringe and gently transfer blood to container containing anticoagulant.

Precautions

1. Take all aseptic precautions.
2. Choose the vein which is straight for at least 2 cm, large enough to insert needle, immovable as far as possible.
3. Always attempt to locate the median cubital vein on either arm before considering alternative veins (cephalic veins and basilic vein).
4. Due to the proximity of the basilic vein to the brachial artery and the median nerve, this vein should only be considered if no other vein is more prominent.
5. To prevent the effects of hemoconcentration from altering test results, the tourniquet should immediately be removed once the blood starts appearing. It will also prevent hematoma formation.
6. Before pricking keep the collection bottle ready.
7. Do not palpate venipuncture site again after cleansing.
8. Immediately transfer blood to anticoagulant containing vial to avoid clotting.
9. Take precautions to prevent hemolysis of blood by:
   - Using clean apparatus and withdrawing blood slowly and not using too fine a needle (Needle used should be less than 22 Gauze)
   - Delivering blood gently into the vial
   - Avoiding frothing during withdrawal of blood and subsequent mixing with the anticoagulant.

Collection of Venous Blood by Using a Vacuum Blood Collection System

Many clinics, hospitals, and labs are collecting blood samples in vacuum blood collection tubes. Blood collection using the vacuum blood collection system produces the best blood samples for analysis by the laboratory because it reduces the incidence of sample hemolysis, contamination, spillage and improper sample volume collection. Thus it improves pre analytical specimen quality as compared to needle and syringe usage. It also facilitates the laboratory information system by lowering specimen identification related errors.

Apparatus

1. Methylated spirit swab
2. Sterile gauze
3. Disposable gloves
4. Tourniquet
5. The Vacuum blood collection system. It consists of:
   - A double-pointed needle: Needle has a sharp point at both ends, one end being

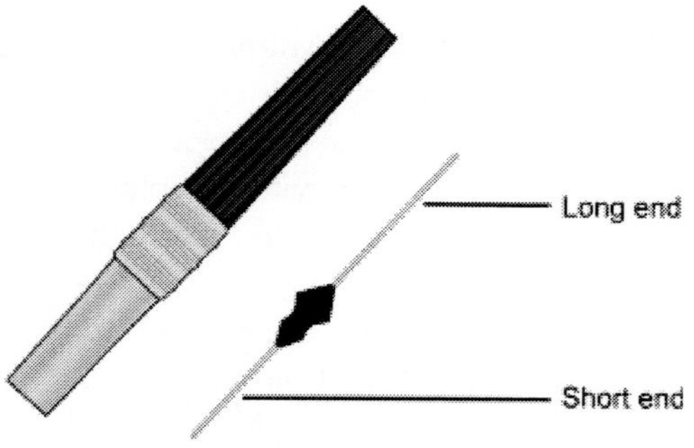

Fig. 2.4: A double-pointed needle

shorter than the other. The long end of the needle is used for penetrating the vein, the shorter end is used to pierce the rubber stopper of the vacuum tube. Usually the needle is covered by a rubber sheath. The sheath makes it possible to draw several tubes of blood by preventing leakage of blood as tubes are changed, this is called a multi-draw. If the short end is not covered with a rubber sheath, it is a single sample needle and only one tube of blood can be collected. There are several sizes of needles available; the size depends on the length and gauge. The needle lengths range from 1 to 1 ½ inches. One inch needles are used for routine venipuncture. The gauge of a needle is a number that indicates the diameter of its lumen. The higher the gauge number of the needle, the smaller is the needle's lumen.

- A plastic holder or adapter: The holder is a plastic cover into which the double pointed needle is screwed. There are different sized holders for adults and pediatric use.
- A series of vacuum tubes: A series of vacuum tubes with rubber stoppers of various colors are used. The colors indicate the type of additives (or no additives)/anticoagulant used.

Vacuum tubes are glass tubes sealed with a partial vacuum inside by rubber stoppers. The air pressure inside the tube is negative, less than the normal environment. After inserting the longer needle into the vein, the tube is pushed into the holder so that the shorter needle pierces the stopper. The difference in pressure between the inside of the tube and the vein causes blood to fill the tube. The tubes are available in various sizes for adult and pediatric use. Adult tubes have volumes of 5, 7, 10 and 15 ml and pediatric tubes are available in volumes of 2, 3 and 4 ml.

Procedure

1. Open needle package but do not remove needle shield.
2. Thread needle onto holder. Select tube or tubes appropriate for the type of sample.

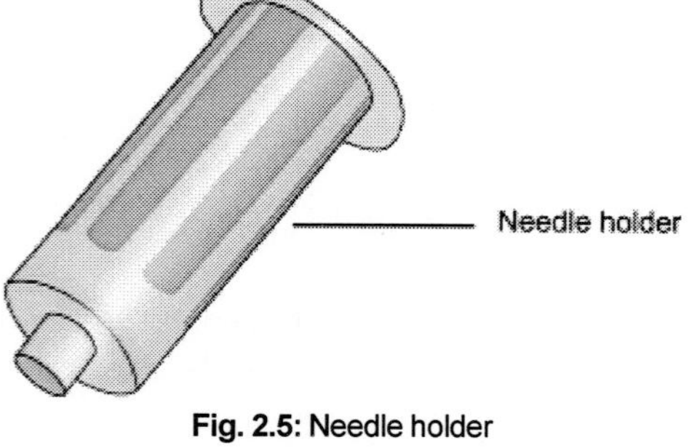

Fig. 2.5: Needle holder

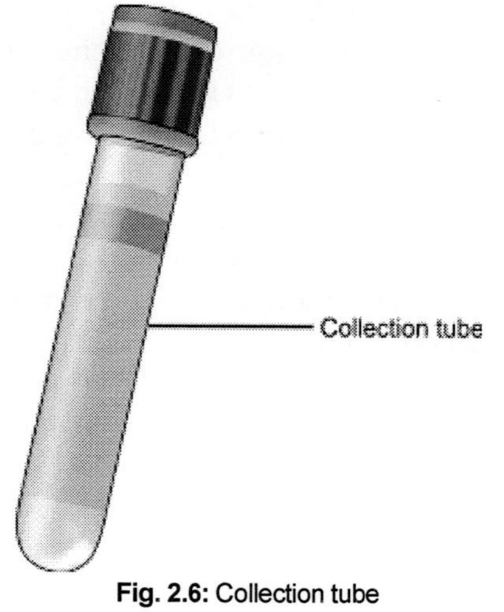

Fig. 2.6: Collection tube

3. Select site for venipuncture by viewing and palpating all available veins of both arms.
4. Apply tourniquet.
5. Clean the puncture site with spirit.
6. Secure patient's arm in a downward position that is stable but yet comfortable for the patient.
7. Remove needle shield.
8. Perform venipuncture as described earlier.
9. Push tube onto holder to puncture diaphragm of stopper.
10. Remove tourniquet as soon as blood appears in tube.
11. When tube is adequately filled remove it from holder.
12. If a multiple sample needle is being used, remove the tube and place a new tube into the holder.
13. Place succeeding tubes in holder, puncturing diaphragm to initiate flow.
14. While each successive tube is filling, invert the previous tube containing additives 8-10 times.
15. As soon as blood stops flowing in the last tube, remove needle from vein. Apply pressure to puncture site with dry, sterile gauze, until bleeding stops.

Precautions

Take all the precaution as described:

1. Tubes that contain anticoagulant should be gently tapped to dislodge any anti-coagulant which may be trapped around the stopper.
2. Do not overfill the collection tube.
3. Tubes without additives are drawn before tubes with additives.
4. Do not shake the tube containing anti-coagulant and blood sample for mixing, just invert it 8-10 times.

WORK SPACE

Q1. What is the difference between plasma and serum?

Q2. Why finger is not squeezed after pricking?

Q3. Why first drop of blood is discarded before taking sample?

Q4. Which finger is preferred for taking capillary blood sample and why?

Q5. Name different tests where capillary blood sample is preferred.

VIVA QUESTIONS

Q1. What are the sites for collecting capillary blood?
Q2. What precautions should be taken before collecting blood sample?
Q3. What precautions are to be taken to prevent hemolysis of venous blood sample?
Q4. Why venous blood sample is not taken in infants and children?
Q5. What is the site for collecting capillary blood in infants?
Q6. What is the advantage of using vacuum blood collection system?

CHAPTER

3

Study of Anticoagulants

OBJECTIVES

After completing practical student should:

- Know the difference betwee *in vitro* and *in vivo* anticoagulants
- Know the commonly used *in vitro* anticoagulants
- Know the mechanism of action of each anticoagulant
- Know the use of different *in vitro* anticoagulant for different blood tests
- Know the recommended quantity of each anticoagulant/unit of blood sample taken
- Be able to identify different anticoagulant vacuum tubes.

INTRODUCTION

Anticoagulants are the chemicals, which prevent blood clotting. They can be used as *In vitro* anticoagulants and *In vivo* anticoagulants.

The concentration of anticoagulant used is very important. If it is inappropriate for volume of blood collected; it may affect cell concentration measures and may also distort cellular morphology. Most often blood is collected directly in commercially prepared negative pressure vacuum tubes which contains the correct concentration of anticoagulant when filled appropriately minimizing the errors. Tubes should be immediately inverted several times to prevent coagulation.

Anticoagulated blood may be stored at 4°C for 24 hours period without significantly altering cell counts or morphology. However, it is preferred to perform hematological analysis as soon as possible after the blood is obtained.

IN VITRO ANTICOAGULANTS

They are used to prevent blood clotting outside body. Anticoagulants are added to blood samples especially when blood is collected by venipuncture and sent to laboratory for investigation. These chemical compounds are also used in medical equipments, laboratory instruments, test tubes and blood transfusion bags.

Commonly used *in vitro* anticoagulants are:

1. Heparin
2. EDTA
3. Sodium Citrate
4. Acid Citrate Dextrose
5. CPD-A (Citrate Phosphate Dextrose-adenine)
6. Oxalate
7. Sodium Flouride.

Heparin

Heparin is present in all the mast cells containing tissues, richest sources are lungs, liver and intestinal mucosa. It was originally isolated from canine liver cells, hence its name (*'hepar'* is Greek for "liver"). Commercial heparin is prepared from ox lungs and pig intestinal mucosa. Heparin is effective as both *in vitro* and *in vivo* anticoagulant. At a concentration of 10-20 IU/ml of blood, it doesn't alter the size or shape of red cells and act as an effective *in vitro* anticoagulant. Green top tube (Sodium Heparin or Lithium Heparin) is used for the collection of heparinized plasma or whole blood.

Mechanism of Action

It acts by facilitating the action of antithrombin III and inhibiting active forms of clotting factors in intrinsic and common pathways (IIa, IXa, Xa and XIa)

Uses

1. It is used for blood gas determination.
2. It is used for pH assay.
3. It is best anticoagulant for osmotic fragility tests.
4. It is used for functional and immunological analysis of leukocytes.

Precautions

1. It should not be used for DLC as it may give a blue color to the ground especially if abnormal proteins are present.
2. It should not be used for total leukocytes count as it causes WBC clumping
3. Heparinized plasma should be stored at room temperature (20-25°C) to minimize intrinsic contact activation at extreme temperature.

EDTA (Ethylenediamine Tetra Acetic Acid Sequestrene/Versene)

EDTA can be used as mono salt (sodium salt, potassium salt, lithium salt), disalt or as trisalt. Sodium and Potassium salts of EDTA are powerful anticoagulants. Dipotassium EDTA is considered best because of its more solubility as compared to sodium and lithium salts. Dilithium salt has an advantage that same sample can be used for chemical investigation but it is less soluble than disodium salt. EDTA is in powder form and used as 1.5 mg/ml of blood. EDTA preserves cellular elements better than oxalates. It is denoted by mauve or lavender top tube.

Mechanism of action

It acts by chelating calcium ions present in blood.

Uses

1. It produces complete anticoagulation with minimal morphological effects on all types of blood cells so it is suitable for all hematological examinations especially for blood cell counts.
2. It is used as an anticoagulant in Wintrobe's method for ESR estimation.

Precautions

1. Tri potassium salts of EDTA causes some shrinkage of RBCs and cause decrease in PCV by 2-3%.
2. If excess of EDTA, i.e. > 2 mg/ml of blood is used it will cause:
    - Shrinkage and degeneration of RBCs
    - Decrease in PCV by 2-3%
    - Increase in MCHC
    - Shrinkage and degeneration of leucocytes
    - Swelling and disintegration of platelets giving false high platelet count as fragments can be confused as individual platelets.

Sodium Citrate

Trisodium citrate 3.2% has been adopted as appropriate concentration by International Committee for Standardization in Hematology. It is in liquid form in light blue top vacuum tube. Because the liquid citrate dilutes the blood, it is important the tube is full so the dilution is properly accounted for.

Mechanism of Action

It prevents coagulation by chelating calcium ions but not as strongly as EDTA.

Uses

1. It is preferred anticoagulant for coagulation studies. Nine volumes of blood are added to one volume of sodium citrate (9 : 1) for coagulation studies (including prothrombin time, partial thromboplastin time).
2. It is also used for ESR estimation by Westergren method. Four volumes of blood are added to one volume of sodium citrate.

Precaution

1. Concentration of 3.8% sodium citrate solution is higher and if used (as done earlier) it may result in falsely lengthened clotting times in calcium dependent coagulation tests (PT and a PTT), with slightly under filled samples and samples with high Hct.

Acid Citrate Dextrose (ACD)

Acid citrate dextrose (ACD) is an important blood anticoagulant and preservative.

It is a solution of citric acid, sodium citrate and dextrose. Yellow top tube denotes ACD. These tubes are used for the collection of whole blood for special tests (e.g. lymphocyte surface markers).

Mechanism of Action

It prevents coagulation by removing calcium ions from blood.

Uses

It is mainly used

1. As an anticoagulant to preserve and store blood in blood banks (Solution A is preferred which comprises of 22.0 g/l trisodium citrate, 8.0 g/l citric acid, 24.5 g/l dextrose). Blood stored in ACD has shelf life of 21 days. Citrate in ACD prevents clotting and dextrose gives energy for sodium potassium pump which maintains volume of RBCs and increases their survival. Some other anticoagulants that allow extended shelf life are preffered over ACD for blood storage. Also owing to the acid pH, 2-3 DGP levels are not well maintained in the solution.
2. For HLA phenotyping.
3. For flow cytometry testing.
4. For Tissue typing.
5. For DNA testing.
6. ACD anticoagulant is believed to be good anticoagulant for leukocyte preservation.
7. It is also used for some special tests like for identification of lymphocyte markers.

Precautions

1. Symptoms attributable to decrease in calcium ions (numbness in fingers, nausea, etc.) may occur after massive administration of ACD preserved blood.
2. ACD is not good medium for rheology studies, as it cause deformability of stored erythrocytes, resulting in bad filterability.

Citrate Phosphate Dextrose-Adenine

It is an anticoagulant solution with phosphate which is associated with higher levels of RBC 2-3 DGP when compared to RBCs stored in ACD. Adenine (maintains nucleotide pool and thus enhance RBC viability) added to CPD extends its shelf-life from 21 to 35 days. Citrate prevents blood clotting and sodium phosphate acts as buffer to control decrease in pH. 63 ml of CPD-A solution is used for 450 ml of collection bag.

Precautions

1. Citrated blood should not be transfused very fast (especially if the liver is damaged) because large amount of citrate if injected too quickly, may lower Ca^{2+} levels in blood to result in tetany and convulsions.

Double Oxalate

It has potassium and ammonium oxalate in the ratio of 2:3. Though each salt can prevent clotting, the mixture of two is used because former alone shrinks RBC while later alone expands them. Double oxalate is prepared by mixing 0.8% potassium oxalate with 1.2% ammonium oxalate. 0.5 ml of this solution is delivered to vial and evaporated to dry in incubator at 37°C. This amount is sufficient for 5 ml of blood. Grey top tubes denote Potassium Oxalate/Sodium Fluoride. This tube contains Potassium Oxalate as an anticoagulant and Sodium Fluoride as a preservative.

Mechanism of Action

It precipitates calcium ions by forming insoluble calcium oxalate complexes and thus removing ionic calcium to participate in clotting.

Uses

It is used for those investigations where volume of blood cells should not be affected, e.g.
1. For estimation of ESR.
2. For estimation of PCV.

Table 3.1: *In vitro* anticoagulants

Anticoagulants	*Mechanism*	*Dose*	*Color of tube tops*	*Used in*
Heparin	inhibit active forms of clotting factors	10-20 IU/ml of blood	Green (Na Heparin)	• Determination of osmotic fragility • Blood gas determination • pH assays • Immunological analysis of WBCs
EDTA	Remove ionic calcium	1.5 mg/ml of blood	Lavender	• Blood counts • ESR determination
Sodium Citrate	Removing ionic calcium	• 9:1 volume for coagulation studies • 4:1 volume for ESR • 1.65 gm/unit of stored blood	Light Blue Black	• Coagulation studies • ESR determination • Blood banks
Acid Citrate Dextrose	Remove ionic calcium	75 ml/unit of blood	Yellow	• Blood banks • Identification of lymphocyte marker • Paternity testing, DNA Studies
Double Oxalate	Chelate calcium	0.5 ml of prepared solution/5 ml of blood	Grey	• ESR determination • PCV estimation

Precautions

1. Don't heat double oxalate mixture at high temperature, high temperature will readily decompose it.
2. Quantity of oxalate added to blood should be accurate because too much oxalate is hypertonic and damages both red and white cells; too little will not prevent clotting.
3. Mono oxalate salts should not be preferred as they alter RBC size.

Sodium Flouride

It is an inhibitor of glycolytic hence mixed with oxalates.

Uses

It is mainly used for preparing blood specimens for plasma glucose estimation.

It is sometimes used as preservative when blood sample has to be stored for few days (a mixture of 10 mg sodium fluoride and 1 mg of thymol acts as anticoagulant as well as preservative).

IN VIVO ANTICOAGULANTS

They are injected in patients to prevent blood clotting in the body. These anticoagulants can be used *in vivo* as a medication for thrombotic disorders (blood clotting inappropriately in the blood vessels), e.g. in primary and secondary prevention of deep vein thrombosis, pulmo-nary embolism, myocardial infarctions and strokes and in those who are predisposed to such like diseases.

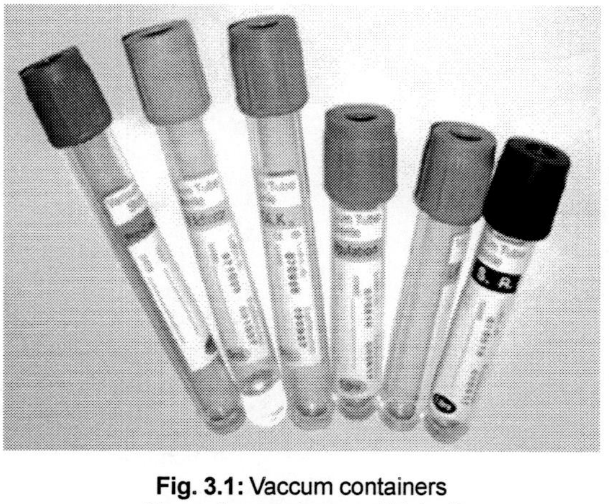

Fig. 3.1: Vaccum containers
(For color version see Plate 1)

Commonly used *in vivo* anticoagulants are:
1. Heparin
2. Warfarin
3. Dicumarol

Heparin

Commercial heparin is extracted from several different animal tissues. Injection of 0.5-1 mg/kg bodyweight causes clotting time to increase from normal 6 minutes to 30 minutes or more. Its actions last for 1.5 hours to 4 hours after its administration. Injected heparin is destroyed by enzyme Heparinase.

Heparin is given intravenously or subcutaneously (Intramuscular injections are avoided because of the potential for forming hematomas also it is degraded when taken orally). Its biologic half-life is one hour so it must be given frequently or as a continuous infusion. However, the use of low molecular weight heparin (LMWH) has allowed once daily dosing, thus not requiring a continuous infusion of the drug. If long-term anticoagul-ation is required, heparin is often used only to commence anticoagulation therapy until the oral anticoagulant warfarin takes effect.

Mechanism of Action

It acts by facilitating the action of antithrombin III and inhibiting active forms of clotting factors IX, X, XI and XII.

Uses

1. It is often used only to commence anti-coagulation therapy until the oral anti-coagulant warfarin takes effect.

2. Heparin is often used during cardiac catheterization, cardio pulmonary by pass surgery and during hemodialysis to prevent clotting.

Side Effects

1. Heparin-induced thrombocytopenia (HITS) is caused which is an immunological response against platelets resulting in the degradation of platelets and thrombocytopenia. This condition is usually reversed on discontinuation, and can generally be avoided with the use of synthetic heparins.
2. Rarer side-effects with chronic use are alopecia and osteoporosis.

Warfarin

By the end of 12 hours of warfarin administration, the coagulation ability of blood decreases to 50% of normal, and by the end of 24 hours it decreases to 20% of normal. Warfarin takes at least 48 to 72 hours for the anticoagulant effect to develop fully, i.e. only after natural consumption of prothrombin and other factors. In cases when any immediate effect is required, heparin must be given concomitantly.

Mechanism of Action

Warfarin competes with vitamin K, which is required by liver for synthesis of clotting factors II, VII, IX and X as well as the regulatory factors protein C, protein S. Other proteins not involved in blood clotting, such as osteocalcin, may also be affected.

Uses

Warfarin is prescribed for thrombosis prophylaxis on long-term basis in:

1. Patients with deep-vein thrombosis.
2. Pulmonary embolism.
3. Atrial fibrillation.
4. Prosthetic heart valves.

Side Effects

1. Hemorrhage – The only common side-effect of warfarin is hemorrhage. Old patients are especially susceptible.
2. Osteoporosis can occur.
3. Purple toe syndrome – This condition is thought to result from small deposits of cholesterol breaking loose and flowing into the blood vessels in the skin of the feet, which causes a blueish purple color and may be painful. It is typically thought to affect the big toe, but it affects other parts of the feet as well, including the bottom of the foot (plantar surface). The occurrence of purple toe syndrome may require discontinuation of warfarin.

Dicumarol

It is a derivative of coumarin that functions as a Vitamin K antagonist (similar to warfarin).

Mechanism

Acts by inhibiting the hepatic synthesis of vitamin K-dependent coagulation factors (prothrombin and factors VII, IX, and X).

Uses

1. It is used as an oral anticoagulant.
2. It is also used in biochemical experiments as an inhibitor of reductases.

WORK SPACE

Q1. Enumerate various clotting factors.

Q2. What is the role of liver in clotting?

Q3. Why double oxalate is preferred over mono oxalate?

VIVA QUESTIONS

Q1. What is the mode of action of EDTA?

Q2. Why EDTA is preferred for venous samples?

CHAPTER

4

Study of Hemocytometry

OBJECTIVES

After completing practical student should:

- Be able to identify different parts of diluting pipettes
- Be able to differentiate between WBC and RBC pipette
- Know uses of each pipette
- Be able to pipette blood and diluting fluid properly
- Know the precautions for pipetting
- Know the dilution employed with each pipette
- Know the dimensions of different squares on counting grid of improved Neubauer chamber
- Be able to identify RBC and WBC squares.
- Be able to charge counting chamber properly
- Know the precautions observed during charging a chamber
- Be able to focus the squares after charging.

INTRODUCTION

Hemocytometry is the procedure of counting the number of cells (RBCs, WBCs and the platelets being counted separately) in a sample of blood. Since the number of blood cells in blood is very high; it is difficult to count them even under microscope. The difficulty is overcome by diluting the blood to a known degree with suitable diluting fluids and then counting cells.

PRINCIPLE

The sample of blood is diluted in a special pipette and is then placed in a capillary space of known capacity (volume) between a counting chamber and a cover slip. The cells spread out in a single layer making their counting easy. Knowing the dilution employed, the number of cells in undiluted blood can then be easily counted.

The result is expressed as so many cells/cu mm of blood (mm^3, μL).

APPARATUS

1. Blood lancet
2. Methylated spirit
3. Sterile gauze
4. Watch glass
5. Microscope
6. Diluting fluids – WBC and RBC diluting fluid
7. Hemocytometer – It includes:
    - Diluting pipette
    - Counting chamber
    - Cover glass/Cover slips – Special cover slips having an optical plane and uniform surface is preferred over ordinary cover slips.

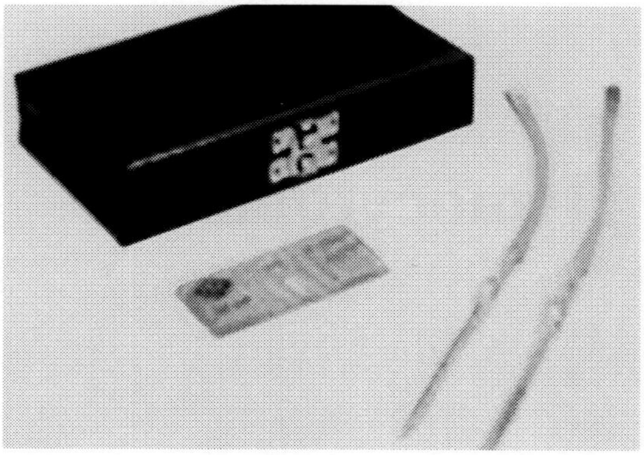

Fig. 4.1: Hemocytometer *(For color version see Plate 1)*

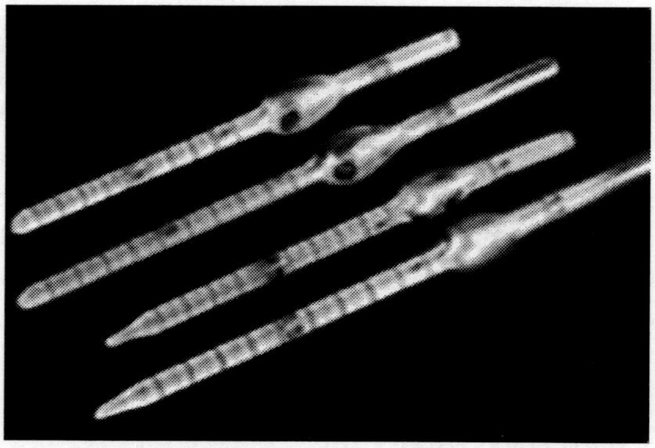

Fig. 4.2: Diluting pipettes *(For color version see Plate 1)*

Diluting Pipettes

Specially designed pipettes are used to dilute blood with a suitable fluid in an accurately known proportion. Each pipette has a long narrow stem (for measuring the blood), which widens into a bulb, which in turn leads to a short stem. There are numbers marked on the stem. These figures indicate relative values (parts)/relative volumes; they don't indicate absolute/definite amounts (volumes) like cu mm/μl.

Mark 0.5 – Half volume
Mark 1 – One volume
Mark11 – Eleven volumes
Mark 101 – Hundred and one volumes

RBC Pipette

I. It has a long narrow stem which is divided into 10 equal parts/graduations but has only 3 markings 0.5 (in middle of stem), 1 (at the junction of stem and bulb), and 101 (immediately above the bulb).

II. The stem has a capillary bore and a well-grounded conical tip. As the capillary bore is narrow the pipette has to be held at 60-70° and it will take a little longer for a suitable drop to form with this pipette. So it is called a slow speed pipette.

III. The stem widens into a bulb. The volume of bulb is 100 times the volume of stem, i.e. the capacity of the bulb is 100 parts (1 to 101 marks). The bulb has a red free-rolling bead in it which:
   - Helps in proper mixing of blood and diluent.
   - Helps in easy identification of the pipette.
   - Tells whether the pipette is dry or not. The bead rolls freely if it is dry.

IV. The bulb narrows to a short stem to which a long narrow soft rubber tube bearing a mouthpiece (red in color) is attached. The tube is long enough to facilitate filling of the pipette by gentle suction. It should have a length of 30-40 cm. It also allows the pipette to be held horizontally so that one can comfortably watch the blood and diluent entering the pipette.

V. On the other end of the tube a red colored mouth piece is attached.

Uses of RBC Pipette

It is used for counting those cells which are more in number so dilution required is more, e.g.

- For RBC counting
- For WBC counting when their number is high as in leukemia
- For spermatozoa counting.

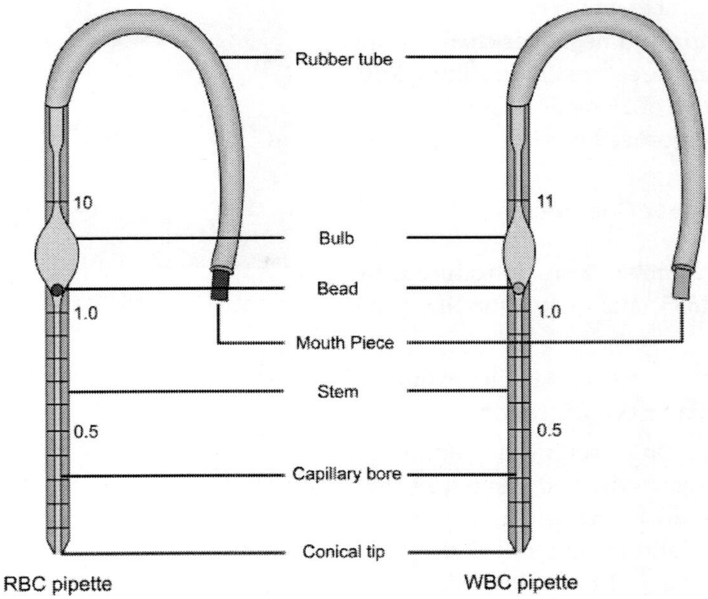

Fig. 4.3: RBC and WBC Pipettes *(For color version see Plate 1)*

WBC Pipette

I. It has a long narrow stem with only 3 markings 0.5 (in middle of stem) and 1 (at the Junction of stem and bulb) and 11 (immediately above the bulb).

II. The capillary bore of the pipette is wider, it is high-speed pipette, a drop will form more quickly at its tip and will be larger. It is to be held at an angle of 10-20°.

III. The bulb is smaller with less capacity (10 parts, i.e. 1 to 11 mark). The volume of bulb is 10 times the volume of stem.

IV. The bulb contains a white bead which has similar functions as that of bead of RBC pipette.

V. The mouthpiece is also white in color.

Uses of WBC Pipette

It is used for counting those cells which are lesser in number, so dilution required is less, e.g.

- For counting white blood cells
- For RBC counting in severe anemia.

Counting Chamber

It is a thick glass slide, ruled with a counting grid. The chamber commonly used for cell counts is Improved Neubauer chamber which has an area of a one sq mm and depth of 0.1 mm. Other counting chambers can also be used. These are:

- Burker chamber which has smaller area and depth as compared to Improved Neubauer chamber.
- Fuchs Rosenthal ruled chamber which has same area but a double depth of 0.2 mm.
- Thomas chamber which has a central circular platform with 1 mm^2 grid having 25 groups of 16 smallest squares (area = 1 mm × 1 mm). 1 mm squares at the corner are absent

- Neubauer chamber which has WBC squares similar to improved neubauer chamber but central 1 mm^2 area has 16 medium RBC squares instead of 25 medium RBC squares as seen in its improved version.

Improved Neubauer Chamber

The counting chamber was introduced by Crammer in 1885 and later modified by Neubauer.

- It is used to obtain a very thin film of fluid of known volume for cellular counts
- It consists of a single solid heavy and thick glass slide which is divided into two central platforms by an H-shaped groove/gutter. The central platform also called the floor piece is wider and 0.1 mm lower than the two lateral platforms/moats
- The two lateral platforms (moats) can support a cover slip, which when in position provide a capillary space (of 0.1 mm depth) between the undersurface of the cover slip and upper surface of floor piece

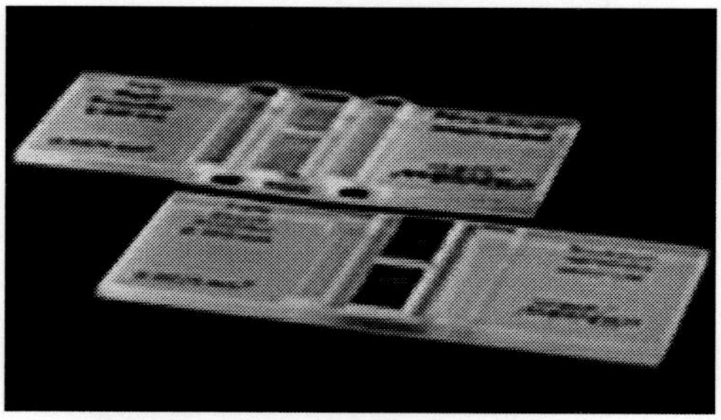

Fig. 4.4: Improved Neubauer chamber
(For color version see Plate 2)

- On the central platform are engraved identical ruled areas called counting grids consisting of squares of different sizes
- The two grids allow RBC and WBC counts to be made simultaneously, if needed duplicate samples can be run
- Each counting grid measures 3 mm × 3 mm.
- This area is divided into 9 large squares each 1 mm × 1 mm
- The 4 large corner squares are lightly etched and are used for counting WBCs
- The large square in the center, which is densely etched, is used for counting RBCs.

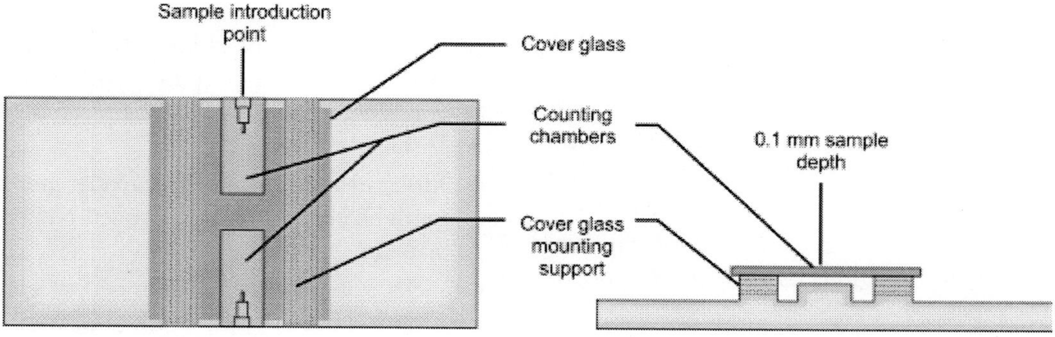

Fig. 4.5: Improved Neubauer chamber

For Total WBC Counting

- Each corner lightly etched WBC square is divided into 16 medium squares.
- Area of one medium square –
  $1/4 \times 1/4 = 1/16\ mm^2$
- Area of 64 (16 × 4) medium squares
  $= 1/16 \times 64$
- Volume of the 64 WBC squares –
  $1/16 \times 64 \times 1/10 = 4/10\ mm^3$

For Total RBC Counting

- The large central densely etched RBC square (1 mm x 1 mm) is divided by means of triple lines/tramlines. (area of one medium square is $1/5 \times 1/5 = 1/25$ sq. mm)
- Each medium sized square is further divided into 16 small squares by single lines. Red cells are counted in the 4 corner medium squares and one central medium square, i.e. 16 × 5 = 80 small squares
- Area of smallest square $1/400\ mm^2$ $(1/20 \times 1/20)$
- Area of 80 smallest squares $1/400 \times 80\ mm^2$
  a. Depth of the chamber - 1/10 mm

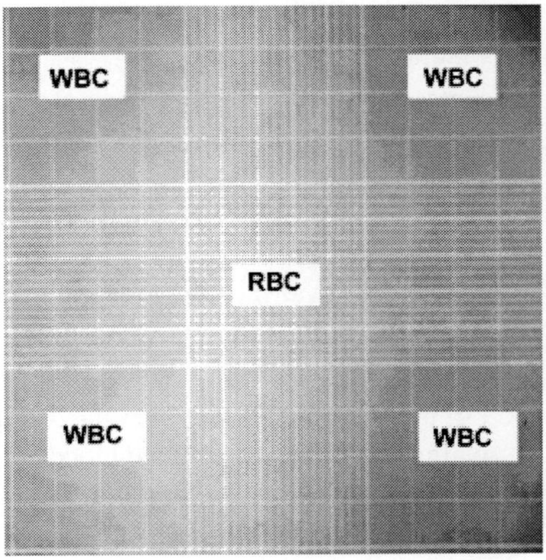

Fig. 4.6: Counting grid of improved Neubauer's chamber

- Volume of the 80 RBC squares = $1/400 \times 80 \times 1/10 = 1/50\ mm^3$.

PROCEDURE

Hemocytometry Includes

Focusing the Counting Grid

1. Examine the grid on each floor piece without the cover slip under low and high magnifications. By adjusting the condenser and the diaphragm find the best combination which shows the grid lines and squares clearly. When properly focused the rulings/lines appear as translucent darkish lines.
2. Under low magnification – One large square (1 mm × 1 mm) is visible in one field, i.e. a group of 16 squares for WBC counting/a group of 25 medium squares for RBC counting.
3. Under high magnification see the grid and the counting area.
4. Focus the WBC and RBC squares.

Pipetting

1. Ensure that the pipette is dry.
2. Collect the diluting fluid in a watch glass.
3. Taking all aseptic precautions, prick the finger tip.
4. Wipe off the first drop of blood.
5. Let another large drop of blood form on the finger tip.
6. Hold the pipette horizontally and dip its tip into the drop of blood. Gently draw blood to the required mark, i.e. 0.5.
7. Wipe the blood sticking to the tip of pipette by non absorbent material. Do not touch the bore of the tip.
8. Immerse the tip of the pipette in the diluting fluid taken in a watch glass and gently suck the diluent to mark 11 for WBC and 101 for RBC counting.

9. Once the diluent has been taken to the appropriate mark, keep the pipette horizontal, so that the fluid does not run out by gravity. Also close the tip of pipette by pressing it against your palm.
10. Mix the contents of the bulb for 2-3 minute by rotating the pipette to and fro with its tip pressed against the palm of left hand and the short stem above bulb between your thumb and first two fingers. The rubber tube can be removed to ease mixing.
11. Place the pipette on a horizontal surface.

Precautions

1. Pipettes should be dry and clean.
2. All precautions are to be taken for finger prick.
3. A large drop of free flowing blood should be allowed to form. If drop of blood is too small, air will enter the pipette along with blood.
4. The tip of pipette should dip into blood drop and it should not be lifted while filling to avoid air bubbles. If the tip is lifted out of the drop, air will enter the pipette along with blood.
5. If any air bubble has entered the pipette discard it and start with a fresh clean and dry pipette.
6. Don't press the tip against skin while pipetting else the bore of tip will get blocked and no blood will enter the stem even if you suck hard at the mouthpiece.
7. Sucking of diluting fluid should not be done very quickly because blood being viscous, if enough time is not allowed; a thick film of blood will remain sticking to the inside of capillary bore giving a significant error.
8. Blood should be sucked exactly up to 0.5 mark. If any excess blood enters, it should be gently tapped on the palm of hand to remove it.
9. Extra blood should not be propelled out or removed by using absorbent material.
10. Tip of the pipette should not be wiped with absorbent material because it will suck the fluid content of blood and that will give false high cell count.
11. Blood should be diluted immediately to prevent clotting.
12. Blood should not be allowed to get into diluent kept in the watch glass and contaminate it as this will affect subsequent cell counts.

Charging the Chamber

1. Clean the counting chamber and cover slip.
2. Place the cover slip on the central platform of the chamber and place it centrally to cover the counting grids and the trenches around them – a process called centering the cover slip.
3. Mix the contents of the bulb of the pipette thoroughly by rolling the pipette between your palms or as described earlier.
4. Discard the first 2 drops of fluid from the pipette.
5. Hold the pipette at an appropriate angle; allow a drop of diluted blood to form at its tip.
6. Quickly but gently place the tip of pipette on the surface of the chamber touching the edge of the cover slip at proper angle.
7. Allow the limited blood to flow under the cover slip by capillary action.
8. Lift pipette quickly as soon as the counting platform is filled with diluted blood.
9. Allow the cells to settle for 2-3 minutes before placing the charged chamber on the stage of the microscope. Counting cannot

be done when cells are moving and changing places due to currents in the fluid.

10. Don't disturb the microscope focus settings.
11. After charging the chamber, place it on the stage of the microscope with its setting intact. Use only the fine adjust-ment screw to focus the cells.

Precautions

1. Ensure that the counting chamber and cover slips are absolutely clean, grease free and dry.
2. The contents of the bulb must be thoroughly mixed before charging otherwise counts are bound to be unreliable.
3. Two drops of fluid must be discarded before charging as the stem of the pipette contains only diluting fluid.
4. The chamber should be charged at one go and not in parts. For this one needs a drop of proper size.

Table 4.1: Non ideal charging

Non ideal charging	*Description*	*Consequence*
Overcharging	If the fluid enters/ over flows into the gutters	Gives false low results
Under charging	If the fluid is insufficient to fill the chamber or if there is any empty space/air bubble	The cells may not be found in the peripheral squares

Note:

* If there is over/under charging, the procedure should be repeated after thoroughly cleaning the chamber and cover slip with soap and water.

* Make sure that the cover slip and chamber are not moist/dirty with grease. This also can cause air bubbles

* Never bring the objective lens down while looking into the microscope as the chamber is likely to be scratched/broken.

5. Chamber should be ideally scharged chamber which is completely filled with diluted blood, neither over nor under charged.

DISCUSSION

Commonly used methods of cell counting are:

1. *Electronic method:* Electronic cell counters are used for counting cells. This method is more accurate. The ease and speed with which cells are counted has increased the practicability of such counts and high level of reproducibility of results has increased its diagnostic value.

   Disadvantages of electronic method are that:
   - It needs costly equipment
   - There can occur calibration error
   - Nucleated RBCs and Platelet clumps are counted as WBCs
   - Giant platelets are counted as RBCs.
2. *Manual method/Hemocytometry:* It is still a necessary procedure
   - For small laboratories which do not have electronic cell counters
   - As reference method for calibration of electronic cell counters.

ERRORS OF HEMOCYTOMETRY

There are two main kinds of errors:

Technical Errors

They can be minimized by care full technique. These are due to inaccurate apparatus and in different technique which includes:

- Bad sampling of blood due to inadequate flow from skin punctures
- Inaccurate pipetting
- Use of badly calibrated pipettes/chambers
- Inadequate mixing

- Faulty filling of pipettes and charging of chambers.
- Careless counting

Inherent Errors

These are due to irregular cell distribution in the counting chamber. They can be minimized by counting large number of cells and making successive counts.

REASONS OF FALSE COUNTS

Falsely high counts occur due to:

1. Blood taken from an area where there is hemoconcentration, e.g. ear lobe.
2. Not removing blood from the outer side of tip of the pipette or if the pipette tip is wiped with any absorbent material.
3. Blood drawn above the mark in the pipette (happens usually when rubber tube is short).
4. Diluting fluid if not taken up to requisite mark.
5. Improper mixing.
6. Uneven distribution in the counting chamber.
7. Presence of extraneous material (yeast or dust etc.).
8. Errors in calculations.

False low counts occur due to:

1. Dilution of blood with tissue fluid due to squeezing.
2. Delay in counting cells. It will effect WBCs more as compared to RBCs (WBCs are reduced by 15% in 24 hours).
3. Less blood drawn.
4. Diluting fluid taken above the requisite mark.
5. Saliva in the mouth piece running into the upper end of the pipette causing dilution.
6. Improper mixing.
7. Uneven distribution in the counting chamber.
8. Errors in calculations.

WORK SPACE

Q1. Give differences between the RBC and WBC pipette.

Difference	*WBC Pipette*	*RBC Pipette*
Calibration marks		
Bore size		
Speed		
Angle at which pipette should be held		
Bulb size		
Dilution achieved		
Bead color		
Color of mouthpiece		

Q2. What are the units of markings on the pipettes?

Q3. What are the uses of WBC and RBC pipettes?

WBC Pipette

RBC Pipette

Q4. Why first two drops of blood are discarded from the pipette before charging the chamber?

Q5. Give dimensions, area and volume of WBC and RBC squares.

Q6. Give features of an ideally charged chamber.

Q7. Calculate the dilution factor in RBC pipette and WBC pipette.

VIVA QUESTIONS

Q1. Name few counting chambers.

Q2. Give the principle of Hemocytometry.

Q3. What are the functions of bead in the pipette?

Q4. How many times blood is diluted in RBC andWBC pipette?

Q5. How do you dilute blood for counting cells?

Q6. How will you level blood if sucked below or above 0.5 mark?

Q7. Why absorbent material is not used for wiping the tip of the pipette?

Q8. What precautions are taken for pipetting and charging chamber?

Q9. What will you do if the chamber is over or under charged?

CHAPTER

5

Determination of Total Erythrocyte Count (RBC)

OBJECTIVES

After completing practical student should:

- Be able to identify RBC pipette, know its uses and the dilution factor employed
- Be able to focus RBC squares of the counting chamber and calculate the volume of RBC squares
- Be able to describe the composition and function of Hayem's fluid
- Be able to pipette the desired amount of blood and Hayem's fluid and charge the chamber properly
- Perform the RBC count and interpret the result
- Give normal RBC count in different age groups.

INTRODUCTION

RBC count is one of the less informative laboratory investigations that may be performed on blood. It is tedious, the margin of error is large, and similar information can be obtained more easily and reliably from Hb estimation and hematocrit estimation. However, it is required to calculate absolute values/ indices. But for the sake of practice, it is desirable to learn the procedure. Also the total RBC count is performed to assess the red cell mass in blood. It is performed if the count is expected to be very high as in polycythemia or low in cases of anemia.

PRINCIPLE

Since the normal RBC count runs in millions, the count is made possible by diluting the blood specimen with the diluting fluid in a red-cell pipette and counting them in the counting chamber. The diluting fluid does not remove the white cells, but allows the red cells to be counted. Knowing the dilution employed, RBC number in undiluted blood is calculated.

APPARATUS

1. Microscope
2. Hemocytometer (RBC diluting pipette and counting chamber)
3. Equipment for a sterile finger prick.
4. Watch glass
5. Cover slip
6. RBC diluting fluid

RBC Diluting Fluid

The ideal fluid for diluting blood

1. Should be isotonic and neither cause hemolysis nor crenation of red cells.
2. It should have a fixative to preserve the shape of RBCs.

3. It should prevent their autolysis so that they can be counted even several hours after diluting the blood if necessary.
4. It should prevent agglutination and should not itself get spoiled on keeping. All these properties are found in Hayem's fluid.

Composition of Hayem's Fluid

1. Sodium chloride 0.5 g
2. Sodium sulphate 2.5 g
3. Mercuric chloride 0.25 g
4. Distilled water 100 ml.

All the components are dissolved thoroughly and filtered several times.

Function of components of hayem's fluid.

1. Sodium chloride maintains osmolarity and provides isotonicity, so that red cells maintain their shape and size.
2. Sodium sulphate prevents aggregation of RBCs; it also acts as an anticoagulant and fixative.
3. Mercuric chloride acts as a preservative. It is antifungal and antibacterial and therefore prevents contamination by growth of microorganisms.

Dacie's fluid, Gower fluid and Isotonic Saline are other diluting agents which can be used for dilution of blood for RBC count.

PROCEDURE

1. Ensure that the improved Neubauer's chamber, coverslip and lenses of the microscope are absolutely clean and the RBC pipette is dry and patent.
2. Take adequate RBC diluting fluid, i.e. Hayem's fluid in a watch glass.
3. Prick the finger under aseptic conditions.
4. Wipe the first drop of blood.
5. Fill the RBC pipette upto 0.5 mark with blood and then suck Hayem's fluid upto 101 mark.

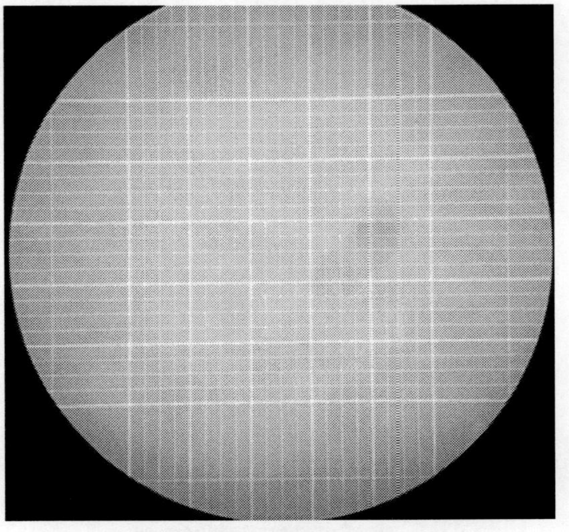

Fig. 5.1: RBC squares under 10X
(For color version see Plate 2)

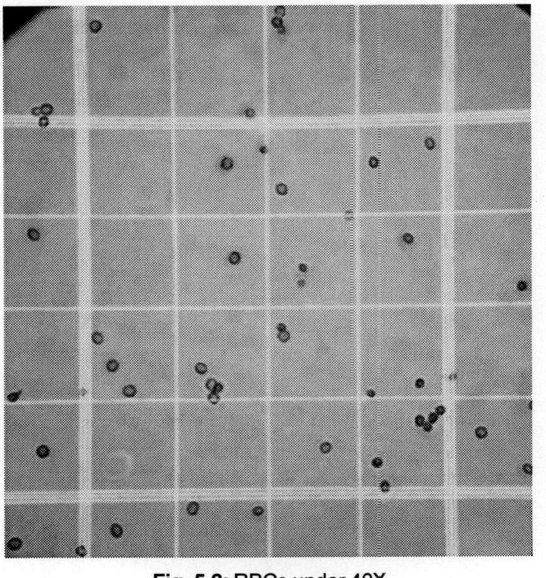

Fig. 5.2: RBCs under 40X
(For color version see Plate 2)

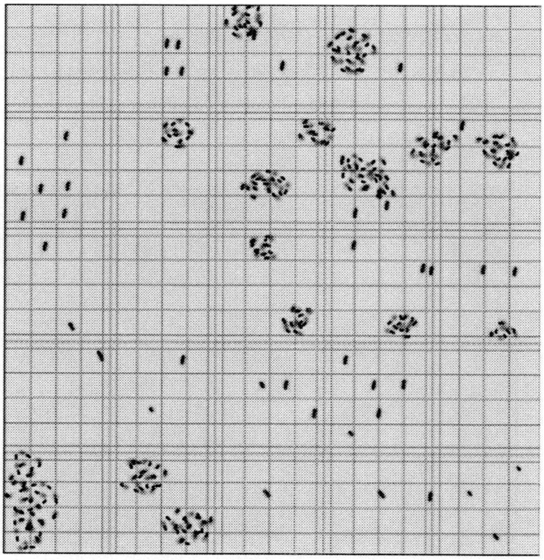

Fig. 5.3: Uneven distribution of cells under 10X

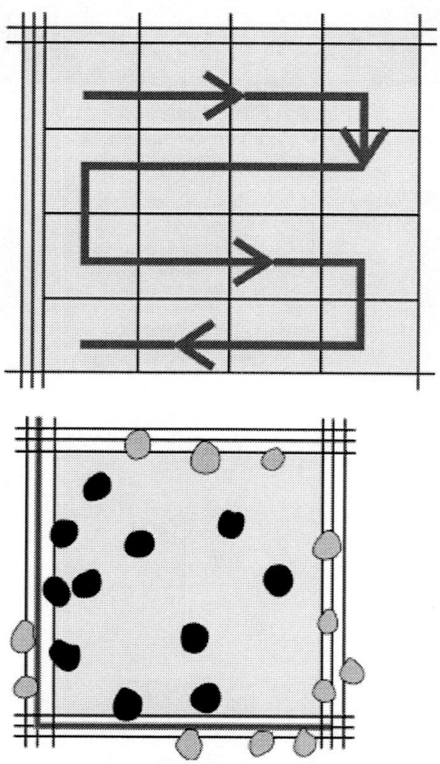

Fig. 5.4: Zig-zag way and 'L' rule of counting cells. Count the cells which are on left and bottom line. *(For color version see Plate 2)*

6. Hold the pipette horizontally and mix the contents of the bulb for 3-4 minutes.
7. Keep the pipette in a horizontal position to prevent any loss of its contents until cell count is performed.
8. Place a clean cover slip on the improved Neubauer's chamber to cover the ruled area on both sides.
9. Examine the chamber under low manification.
10. Focus the RBC counting area of the counting grid.
11. Without distrubing imcroscope settings remove the chamber from the microscope. Place it on the work table.
12. Before charging, remix the contents of the RBC pipette.
13. Discard the first 2 drops of fluid from the pipette as this is cell-free.
14. Allow a small drop of fluid to form at the tip of the pipette and bring it gently in contact with the edge of the cover slip.
15. Since the RBC pipette is a slow speed pipette it will need to be kept at an angle of 60-70° while charging the chamber.
16. The fluid will be drawn into the chamber by capillary action.
17. Ensure that it is an ideally charged chamber.
18. Move the chamber onto the microscope stage and fine focus the RBC squares.
19. Wait for 3-4 minutes for the cells to settle down because they cannot be counted when they are moving and changing their position due to currents in the fluid.
20. Check whether the cells are uniformly distributed or not. If they are unevenly distributed, i.e. bunched at some places and scanty at others, the chamber has to be washed, dried and recharged.
21. Focus the RBC squares under high power objective and count the cells.

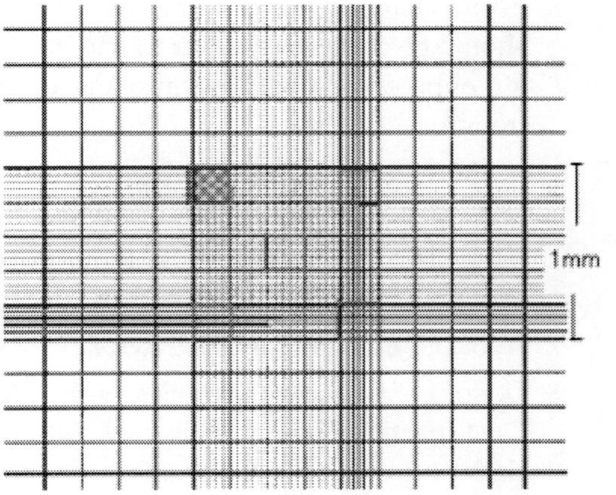

Fig. 5.5: RBC counting squares outlined in pink
(For color version see Plate 2)

COUNTING OF CELLS

1. Count the cells in the 5 medium sized-RBC squares, i.e. 4 on each corner and one in the centre (as shown in Fig. 5.5).
2. In each medium square first count cells in the upper 4 horizontal small squares then come down to the next row of small squares and count cells is squares from right to left. Then count the 3rd row from left to right and 4th row from right to left.
3. Care should be taken not to count the same cell twice.
4. Cells lying within a square are to be counted in that square.
5. Count the cells present on the left and lower lines of the square – the "L rule" for counting (as shown in Fig. 5.4).
6. Ignore those on the right and upper lines.
7. In squares bordered by triple lines, the middle line is assumed to be the boundary of the square (as shown in Fig. 5.4).
8. Enter the observations in your workspace.
9. Count the cells in all 5 medium RBC squares.

CALCULATIONS

Calculation of Dilution Factor

1. 0.5 parts of blood and 100.5 parts of RBC diluting fluid are present in the pipette.
2. As blood get mixed with the diluting fluid only in the bulb of the pipette and diluting fluid in the stem of the pipette does not take part in dilution.

So 0.5 part of blood mixes with 99.5 parts of diluting fluid in the bulb of the pipette to form (0.5 + 99.5) = 100 parts of the solution.

Hence the dilution factor is:

$$\frac{\text{Final volume achieved (100 parts)}}{\text{Original volume taken (0.5 parts)}} = 200$$

Calculation of the Volume of Fluid Examined

Area of 1 medium size square is
$= 1/5 \times 1/5 = 1/25\ mm^2$

Area of 5 medium sized squares
$= 5 \times 1/25 = 1/5\ mm^2$

Depth of the chamber = 1/10 mm

Volume of the fluid in 5 RBC squares $1/5 \times 1/10 = 1/50\ mm^3$

Calculation of the RBC Count

If N is the no. of cells counted in the 5 RBC squares, i.e. in 1/50 mm^3 volume of diluted blood; Then cells in 1 mm^3 volume of diluted blood will be N × 50.

Therefore cells in one mm^3 of undiluted blood
= N × 50 × 200 (Dilution factor)
= N × 10,000

Result

The result is expressed as "x" million cells/mm^3

Sources of Error

Despite all precautions the degree of error with this method is about 15 - 20%.

This is because of:

1. *Pipette Error:* Inaccuracy of graduations on the pipette, improper volume measurement, improper method of filling of blood and diluent and their mixing.
2. *Chamber Error:* The process of improper charging may introduce an error. The counting grid and depth of chamber may not be accurate.
3. *Field Error:* The distribution of cells in the grid may not be uniform.
4. *Experimental error:* Since the multiplication factor is 10,000, an error in counting of even 1 RBC will cause a variation of total RBC count by 10000/cu mm of blood. Therefore,
   - The test should be carried out as meticulously as possible
   - More number of cells can be counted and counting can be done on both sides of the chamber. The average of these can be taken. This reduces error
   - Taking repeated samples of blood, counting cells in each and taking their mean value can eliminate pipette error. But this is hardly of any practical value.

Precautions

1. Observe all precautions for finger pricking.
2. The pipette, chamber and cover slip should be clean and dry.
3. Follow all precautions for pipetting.
4. Follow all precautions for charging of chamber.
5. While charging the chamber the platform should be completely covered and have no air bubbles or overflow into the central trough.
6. If there is over/under charging, wash, clean, dry, and recharge the chamber.
7. If the distribution of cells is not uniform (as shown in Fig. 5.3), discard and recharge.
8. Avoid counting of same cell twice.
9. Donot confuse dust particles with RBCs. Dust particles are angular, of different sizes and colors. RBCs on other hand are round discs, of uniform size and lighter in the center.

NORMAL RANGE OF RBCs/CU MM OF BLOOD

In males: 4.75 - 6.0 millions/mm^3 of blood

In females: 4 - 5.5 millions/mm^3 of blood

DISCUSSION

Polycythemia

- Increase in RBC count more than the normal range
- Dilution may have to be increased for counting RBCs in polycythemia.

Anemia

- It is defined as decrease in RBC count or Hb concentration
- Dilution may have to be decreased for counting RBCs in anemia.
- The 1 mark is used for pipetting blood in conditions of severe anemia where more blood is taken for dilution giving a dilution of 1 in 100.

Fate of WBC in RBC Count

WBCs are not lysed by RBC diluting fluid but as the normal ratio of RBC: WBC is 700 : 1 and the RBCs counted in 5 squares are usually less than 700, so hardly any WBC will be seen in the field. Any occasional WBC (may be 1 in 600 - 700 RBCs) if seen will be grayish, nucleated, refractive and granular, and larger than RBC. It should not be counted with RBC as it will increase the count by 10,000/mm^3.

Other Uses of RBC Pipette

- It is used for counting WBC in leukemia where leukocytes are present not in thousands but in lakhs or millions/mm^3 of blood. There also blood is sucked upto mark 1 in RBC pipette and then diluted to 101 mark giving a dilution of 1 in 100.
- The RBC pipette is also used for sperm count and platelet count.

Conditions That Alter Total RBC Count

Decreased RBC Count is Seen in:

1. Physiological: Pregnancy, children, and women.
2. Pathological: Anemia and other conditions like posterior pituitary tumors.

Increased RBC Count is Seen in:

1. Physiological: High Altitude (due to hypoxia), newborns, excessive sweating.
2. Pathological: Polycythemia rubra Vera, emphysema, congenital heart disease and conditions that produce hemoconcentration like severe diarrhea and vomiting.

WORK SPACE

OBSERVATIONS

Date Age

Name Sex

A

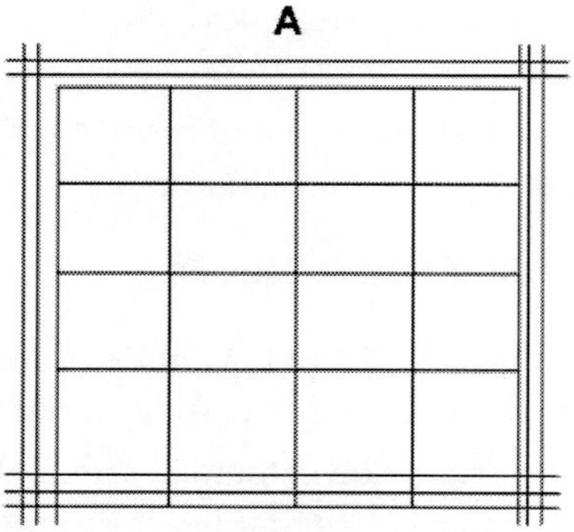

Upper right square

B

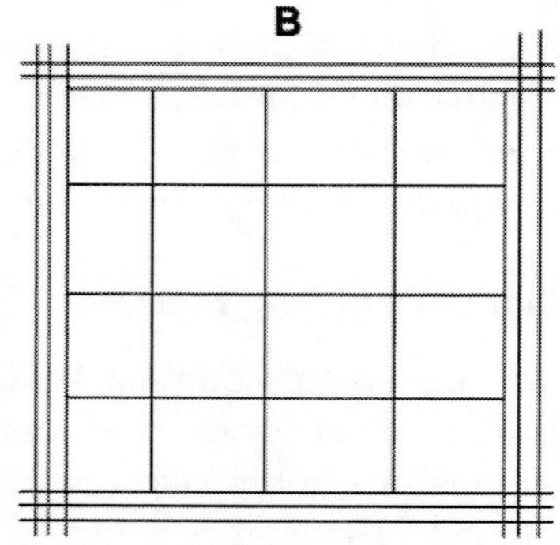

Upper left square

C

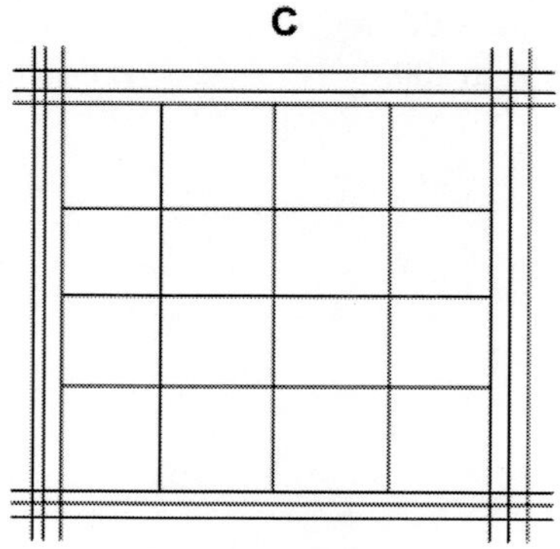

Central Square

D

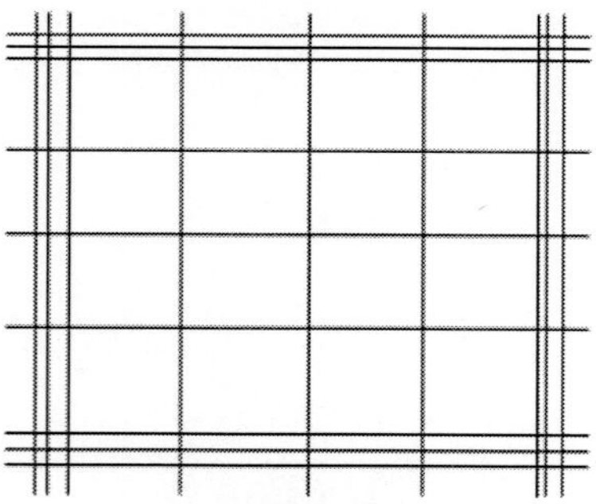

Lower Right Square

E

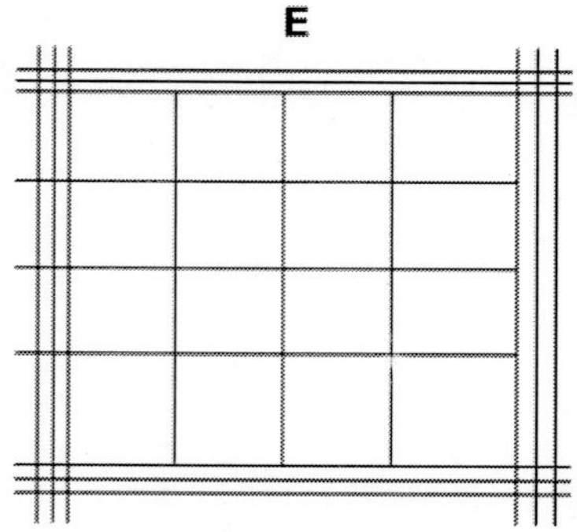

Lower left square

Total cells in A + B + C + D + E =

Calculations

Result

Inference

ANSWER THESE QUESTIONS

Q1. Give the composition and function of each component of Hayem's fluid.

Q2. How is dilution factor calculated in RBC pipette?

VIVA QUESTIONS

Q1. Name few diluting fluids for counting RBCs.

Q2. What is the function of red bead in RBC pipette?

Q3. How will you differentiate RBC pipette from WBC pipette?

Q4. What is the dilution obtained with RBC pipette?

Q5. Why is blood diluted 200 times in RBC counting?

Q6. Can RBC pipette be used for counting WBCs?

Q7. Besides counting RBCs what are the other uses of RBC pipette?

Q8. Why first two drops of the solution are discarded from the pipette before charging the chamber?

Q9. What happens to WBCs in RBC count?

Q10. What is the normal RBC count?

Q11. Give physiological conditions which alter RBC count?

Q12. Why RBC count is more in males than females?

Q13. Why RBC count is more at high altitude?

CHAPTER

6

Determination of Total Leukocyte Count

OBJECTIVES

After completing the practical student should:

- Be able to identify WBC pipette and differentiate it from RBC pipette.
- Know the composition of Turk's fluid and function of each component of turk's fluid.
- Be able to pipette requisite amount of turk's fluid and blood in WBC pipette.
- Know the dilution employed in WBC counting.
- Be able to charge the counting chamber.
- Be able to identify WBC squares, calculate their volume, describe the basis of calculation of WBC count.
- Perform a WBC count.
- Interpret the result.

INTRODUCTION

TLC is a part of routine laboratory hematological investigation to assess the nature and severity of infection, extent of disease and body's defence capabilities. TLC alone could be diagnostic in some cases but it is more frequently done along with DLC. There are two methods of determining TLC.

- *Electronic automated method:* It is more accurate and uses electronic cell counters
- *Manual method:* It is less accurate method but it is widely used in undeveloped countries because of lesser cost.

PRINCIPLE

A sample of blood is diluted with diluting fluid, which lyses RBCs, platelets and stains nuclei of WBCs. Cells are then counted in hemocytometer under microscope. With the knowledge of volume of fluid examined and dilution done, the result is given as number of WBCs/cu mm of undiluted whole blood.

APPARATUS

1. Equipment for sterile finger prick
2. Watch glass
3. Microscope
4. Cover slip
5. Hemocytometer – WBC pipette and modified Neubauer's chamber.
6. Turk's fluid – It is used as diluent. Each 100 ml of Turk's fluid contains:
   i. Glacial acetic acid (2 ml of 1-2%)
   ii. Gentian violet stain (1 ml of 1%)
   iii. Distilled water.

Functions of Constituents of Turk's Fluid

Glacial acetic acid: It hemolyzes RBCs. The remnants of RBC membrane are faintly visible under microscope and are called ghost cells. Glacial acetic acid is preferred over any other hemolytic agent because any weak acid used in its place would take inordinately long time to lyse RBCs and strong acid if used will damage WBCs.

Glacial acetic acid being pure acetic acid imparts shine/halo to WBCs. This refractility of WBCs differentiates them from dust particles which are nonrefractile, opaque and are of different sizes.

Gentian violet stain: It stains nuclei of WBCs. Cytoplasm is not stained.

Distilled water: It is used as solvent.

PROCEDURE

It involves:

Pipetting

1. Ensure that the Neubauer's chamber, cover slips and lenses of the microscope are absolutely clean and the WBC pipette is dry and patent.
2. Take adequate amount of Turk's fluid in a watch glass.
3. Prick the fingertip under aseptic conditions.
4. Wipe the first drop of blood.
5. Fill the WBC pipette upto 0.5 mark with blood and then suck Turk's fluid upto 11 mark.
6. Hold the pipette horizontally and mix the contents of the bulb for 3-4 minutes by rolling it between your palms.
7. Keep pipette aside in a horizontal position for 8-10 minutes. This time is given for membrane lysis of RBCs, WBCs and platelets.

Charging

1. Place a clean cover slip on the counting chamber to cover the ruled area on both sides.
2. Examine the chamber under low power and focus WBCs square of the counting grid.
3. Remove the chamber from the microscope stage and place it on the worktable.
4. Mix the contents of the WBC pipette again and discard the first two drops of fluid from the pipette (as it is cell free).
5. Allow a small drop of fluid to form at the tip of the pipette and bring it gently in contact with the edge of the cover slip at an angle 0f 10-20°.
6. The fluid will be drawn into the chamber by capillary action. Ensure that it is an ideally charged chamber.

Focussing

1. Wait for 3-4 minutes for the cells to settle down (because they cannot be counted when they are moving and changing their position due to currents in the fluid).
2. Put the charged chamber on the microscope stage.
3. Without disturbing the microscope settings, bring WBC squares in the view.
4. Start with low power and focus the grid lines. Continuously rack microscope up and down with fine adjustment screw. Lines will come into and go out of focus alternatively. Under low power objective you will see 16 squares of one large corner square in one field.
5. Try to identify the Leukocytes. They appear as shiny dark dots with a halo around them. Dark dots represent stained nucleus of Leukocytes.
6. Check the pattern of distribution of cells if they are unevenly distributed (i.e. bunched at some places and scanty at others), the chamber has to be washed, dried and recharged.

Counting of Cells

1. If the cells are uniformly distributed, count the cells in the 4 WBC squares, i.e. $16 \times 4 = 64$ small squares
2. Continuously rack the microscope while counting to avoid missing any cell and to appreciate 3-dimension of cells.
3. First count cells in the upper 4 horizontal squares then come down to the next row

and count cells in squares from right to left. Then count the 3rd row from left to right and 4th row from right to left.

4. Count the cells present on the left and lower lines of the square. Follow The "L rule" for counting. Ignore those on the right and upper lines.
5. Cells lying within a square are to be counted in that square. Care should be taken not to count the same cell twice.
6. Add up the number of cells in each of the 4 blocks of squares.
7. Enter the observations in the given workspace.

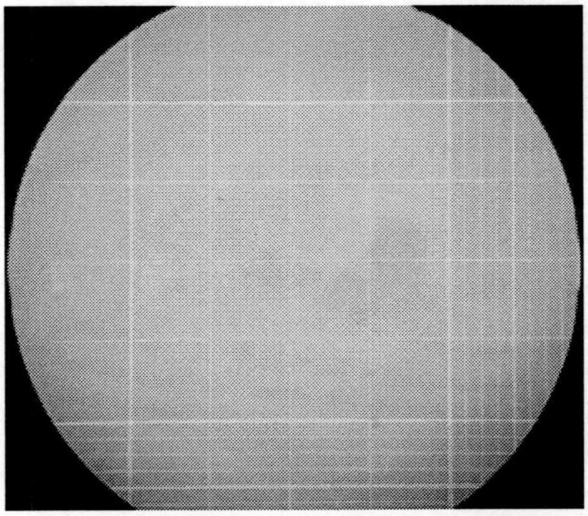

Fig. 6.1: WBC squares under microscope
(For color version see Plate 3)

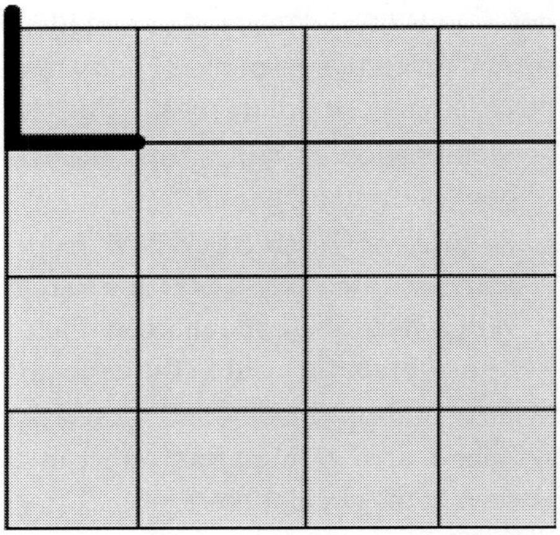

Fig. 6.2: "L rule" of counting cells

CALCULATIONS

Calculation of Dilution Factor

1. 0.5 parts of blood and 10.5 parts of WBC diluting fluid are present in the pipette.
2. Blood gets mixed up with the diluting fluid only in the bulb of the pipette (1 part of the diluting fluid which remains in the stem of the pipette does not take part in dilution).
3. So 0.5 part of blood mixes with 9.5 parts of diluting fluid in the bulb of the pipette to form (0.5 + 9.5) = 10 parts of the solution.
4. Hence the dilution factor is:

$$\frac{\text{Final volume achieved (10 parts)}}{\text{Original volume taken (0.5 parts)}} = 20$$

Calculation of the Volume of Fluid Examined

Area of 1 WBC squares = $1 \times 1 = 1\ mm^2$
Area of 4 WBC squares = $4 \times 1 = 4\ mm^2$
Volume of 4 WBC squares = $4 \times 1/10$
= $4/10\ mm^3$

Dilution factor = 20
Cells in 4/10 cu mm volume of diluted blood = n
Cells in 1 mm^3 of diluted blood = $n \times 10/4$
Cells in mm^3 of undiluted blood
= $n \times 10/4 \times$ Dilution factor
= $n \times 10/4 \times 20$
= $n \times 50$

PRECAUTIONS

1. Observe all the aseptic precautions.
2. The apparatus used should be clean and dry.
3. Take all precautions for blood sample collection and hemocytometry.
4. Pipette should be held in horizontal position while mixing to prevent centri-fugation of Leukocytes towards the ends of the pipette.
5. After mixing the blood with Turk's fluid, sufficient time for hemolysis of RBCs should be given.

6. Before charging chamber pipette contents should be mixed again and first two drops should be discarded.
7. Once the chamber is charged complete the counting as early as possible before the fluid begins to dry.
8. Always follow the "L rule" for counting to avoid counting the same cell twice.
9. Microscope should be continuously racked while counting to avoid missing any cell sticking to the under surface of cover slip or confuse dust particle for WBC.
10. Don't confuse WBCs with dust particles which are opaque, of varying sizes and shapes, often angular with no halo around them. They may be brown, black or yellow in color.

SOURCES OF ERROR

Technical Errors

1. Improper volume measurements of either blood or diluents.
2. Use of defective pipette (broken tips).
3. Improper charging (over/under).
4. Improper counting.
5. Wrong calculation.

Inherent Errors

1. Errors of visual count.
2. Mistaking dust particles or clumped RBC debris for WBCs. This error can be decreased by doing 2nd count on opposite side of counting grid.
3. Error due to non uniform distribution.

NORMAL COUNT

Adults	–	4000 - 11,000/cu mm
Children	–	5000 -15,000/cu mm
Newborns	–	10000-25, 000/cu mm
Infants	–	6000 - 18,000/cu mm

DISCUSSION

Leukocyte Pool in Body

There are two pools of Leukocyte in body:

Circulating pool: It includes all the Leukocytes freely moving in the circulation.

Marginal pool: It includes Leukocytes which are sticking to the endothelial walls of closed capillaries, venules, small veins, and sinusoids.

There is a rapid exchange between these pools. For each mature WBC in the circulation there are 50-100 such cells held in the bone marrow which acts as reservoir of Leukocytes. From the bone marrow cells enter circulation, remains there for 8-10 hours and then enter tissues. In the tissues they remain for few days then die.

Variation in WBC Count

WBCs constitute major defense system of the body against invasion of bacteria, viruses, fungi, toxins and foreign agents. Their number in body is kept remarkably constant in health but increase or decrease is seen in many diseases.

Leukocytosis

The term is used when there is increase in the number of WBCs >11000/cu mm of blood. It is a normal protective response of body to various types of stresses. It occurs mostly due to:

1. Mobilization of WBCs from the marginal pool to circulating pool.
2. Release of reserved WBCs from bone marrow. If leucocytosis is due to release of WBCs from the bone marrow there won't be any immature cell in the circulation.
3. Increased production and release from the bone marrow. Immature cells can also be seen in the circulation.

Physiological Causes of Leukocytosis

1. Newborns and infants.
2. Physical exercise: Dynamic circulation in exercise will disrupt the marginated pool of WBCs.
3. Meals: Increased metabolism will improve circulation and will disturb marginated pool of WBCs.
4. Pregnancy: Exact cause is not known. It may be because of the effect of hormones on leucopoiesis.
5. Parturition: Combined effect of tissue injury, hemorrhage, and severe exertion will lead to leukocytosis.
6. Menstruation
7. Exposure to sun or increased temperature will also disturb marginal pool to cause increase in Leukocyte count.

Pathological Causes of Leukocytosis

1. Acute bacterial infection
2. Chronic Bacterial infection
3. Tissue Injury like infraction, burns and surgery
4. Hemorrhage
5. Neoplasia
6. Inflammatory disorder
7. Steroid therapy

Leukopenia

Decrease in WBCs count < 4000/cu mm is called Leukopoenia. Causes are:

1. Severe cold.
2. Typhoid.
3. Paratyphoid.
4. Viral infection like mumps, influenza and AIDS.
5. Sepsis: Due to consumption of normal neutrophils which exceeds production.
6. Repeated X-ray exposure.
7. Replacement of hemopoietic tissue by neoplastic infiltration.
8. Acute leukemia or pre-leukemic stage, lymphoma, multiple myeloma, myelofibrosis, and aplastic anemia.
9. Chemotherapy.
10. Use of drugs like Chloramphenicol, Sulphonamides, Aspirin, Penicillins, Cyclosporine, Phenytoin etc.
11. Malnutrition – General malnutrition and specific deficiency of Vitamin B12 and Folic acid.

Leukemia

It is a cancerous disease of blood (WBCs) forming tissue (bone marrow and lymphoid tissue). There occur uncontrolled production and release of mature and immature WBCs into the circulation. It can be myeloid (involving neutrophils) or lymphatic (involving lymphocytes), the raised count can be from 40,000-50,000 to few lakhs/cu mm.

Leukostasis

When the leukocyte count goes above 100,000/cu mm, white cell thrombi may form in the brain, lungs, heart, etc.

Leukemoid Reaction

It is an extreme elevation of TLC above 50,000/cu mm seen in severe chronic infections, severe hemolysis or malignant growths. Both immature and mature cells are seen.

WORK SPACE

Date Name

Sex Age

OBSERVATIONS

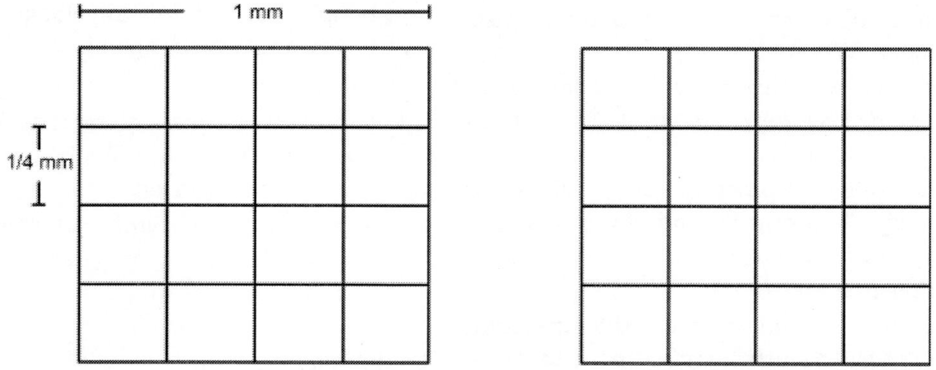

A (Left upper square) B (Right upper square)

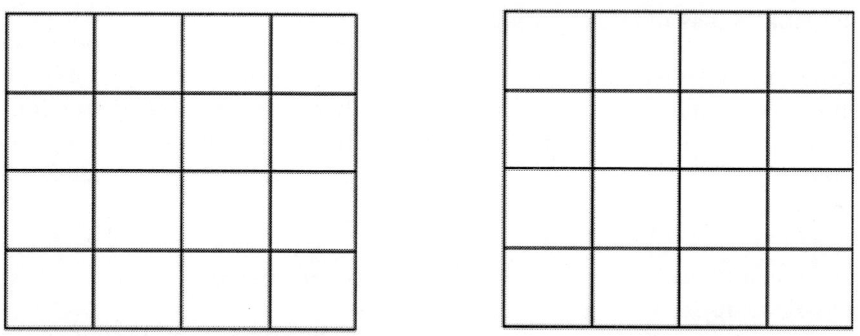

C (Left lower square) D (Right lower square)

Total cells A + B + C + D =

Calculations

Result

Inference

ANSWER THESE QUESTIONS

Q1. List the uses of WBC pipette.

Q2. Calculate dilution factor for determination of TLC.

Q3. Give composition and function of each component of Turk's fluid.

Q4. Why red cells are not seen when counting Leukocytes?

Q5. Can any other agent be used to lyse RBCs?

VIVA QUESTIONS

Q1. What are the units of markings on the WBC pipette?
Q2. What is the function of bead in the pipette?
Q3. How will you differentiate WBCs from dust particles?
Q4. Enumerate differences between RBC pipette and WBC pipette.
Q5. Why the bulb in WBC pipette is smaller than RBC pipette?
Q6. Why acetic acid used in Turk's fluid should be Glacial?
Q7. What is the function of Leukocytes?
Q8. Name the few causes of leukocytosis.
Q9. Give conditions in which leucopoenia is seen.
Q10. What is Leukemia? How will you differentiate it from Leukocytosis?
Q11. What is Leukemoid reaction?
Q12. What are Ghost cells?
Q13. In which condition RBC pipette is used for counting WBCs?

CHAPTER

7

Preparation and Examination of Peripheral Blood Smear

OBJECTIVE

After completing the practical student should:

- Know the importance of peripheral blood film examination
- Know the precautions observed for preparing blood smear
- Be able to form an ideal smear
- Know the features of an ideal blood smear
- Know the composition of Leishman's stain and function of its each component
- Be able to stain smear ideally without under or overstaining it
- Identify different types of leukocytes, i.e. neutrophils, eosinophils, basophils, lymphocytes and monocytes
- Be able to differentiate a neutrophil from an eosinophil and a large lymphocyte from a monocyte
- Draw illustrative diagrams of all types of leukocytes.

INTRODUTION

Many hematological and other medical disorders can be diagnosed by careful examination of stained blood film.

- It provides information about the morphology of red cells, platelets and leukocytes
- It can be used to determine differential leukocyte count
- It can also be used to detect presence of various parasites like malarial and filarial parasite
- Smear can be retained and preserved as an original record to evaluate the progress of patient.
- Sex of a person can also be determined by identifying the presence of Barr body in neutrophil (it requires the use of special stains).

Examination of smear is done in following steps:

1. Preparation of peripheral smear.
2. Fixing and staining the smear.
3. Examining the stained smear under microscope.

PREPARATION OF PERIPHERAL BLOOD SMEAR

A blood smear is made by 3 methods:

1. Glass slide method/wedge method
2. Cover glass method
3. Centrifugal method

Glass slide Method/Wedge Method

It is the most commonly used method.

Principle

For making a thin film, a drop of blood is spread on glass slide.

Apparatus

1. Clean, grease-free slides: It is essential to use clean, dry, dust-free slides; remember that grease and residual detergent are equally liable to spoil a blood film.
2. Spreader: Select a glass microscope slide with at least one smooth end. Each spreader can be used repeatedly provided that the spreading edge remains smooth. The edge must be wiped carefully and dried before and after each use, and the slide must be discarded if the spreading edge becomes chipped.
3. Lancet.
4. Cotton swab.
5. Methylated spirit.

Procedure

1. Prick fingertip under all aseptic conditions. Discard first drop of blood.
2. Let a good size blood drop form on the tip spontaneously.
3. Place a small drop of blood in the center at one edge of slide 1 cm from one end.
4. With left hand, support the slide with thumb and finger on the table.
5. Take the spreader slide (in thumb and index finger of right hand) at an angle of 30° in front of drop. Pull it backwards, to touch the edge of blood drop; blood will automatically spread along the full width of spreader (or move a little side to side). Hold it there.
6. Steady the slide first with left hand and with light even pressure (of right hand) at 30°, move spreader forward in a single smooth fairly fast gliding motion pulling the blood behind in a thin smear. (Spreading of smear should take 1/2 sec only).
7. Dry the film by waving in air.
8. Examine with naked eye. Observe color, thickness, length and quality of smear to select good smear for staining.
9. Make as many trial slides as possible to get good smears. Practice and keep best slide for staining.

Precautions

1. Slides should be clean (preferably new) and grease-free, else blood will not stick to these areas.
2. Do not touch the skin while applying blood drop to slide (to avoid epidermal cell/sweat deposition on the slide).
3. Spreader should have smooth edge otherwise striations will appear on smear and leukocytes may accumulate at the edges and tail.
4. Spreader should be at 30° angle and pressure should be slight and uniform while spreading.
5. Spread blood immediately, any delay will lead to clumping of cells and granular appearance of smear. The spreader must not be lifted off the slide until the last trace of blood has been spread out; with a correctly sized drop the film should be about 3 cm in length.
6. It is important that the film of blood finishes at least 1 cm before the end of the slide.
7. Film should be air dried by waving in air immediately after spreading. Delay will lead to clumping, crenation or distortion of red cells in a damp atmosphere as water slowly evaporates from blood plasma on slide area due to gradual increase in concentration of salts.
8. Mark smeared surface with a glass marking pencil.
9. Stored blood should not be used for smear preparation. Anticoagulated blood standing for more than 1-3 hours at room temperature will cause appearance of small vacuoles in cytoplasm and separation of nuclear lobes.

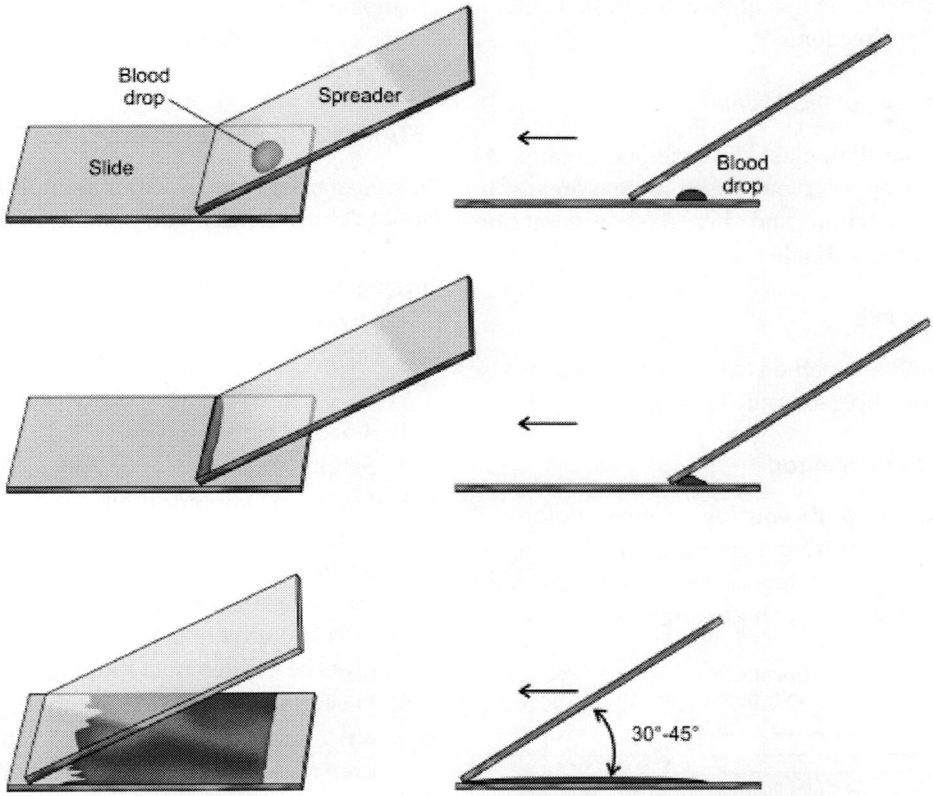

Fig. 7.1: Method of smear preparation *(For color version see Plate 3)*

Features of Ideal Blood Film

1. Film should occupy middle 2/3 of slide length covering almost entire width.
2. It should be buff colored.
3. It should be tongue-shaped (broad at head, tapering at other end) but should not have tails.
4. It should not have any vacant area or striations.
5. It should have uniform thickness. A properly made film/smear should be one cell thick throughout (on observing under microscope). In very thin film neutrophils, monocytes accumulate at edges and tail. In thick films, red cells are not clearly visible. The thickness of the film can be regulated by varying the—
   - Size of blood drop
   - The pressure and speed of spreading (faster rate will lead to thin film and slower rate will lead to thick films.)
   - Angle at which it is held (larger angle: thicker film).
   - With anemic blood the correct thickness is achieved by using a wider angle and, with polycythemic blood, the angle should be narrower.

Cover Slip Method

A drop of blood is placed over a cover slip, which is topped over with another cover slip in a crosswise fashion so that its corners form a star. After a moment when the drop of blood has spread over, the two of them are pulled apart in opposite direction.

Advantages of this Method

It is better than glass slide method because the small drop of blood used here spreads by capillary action and hence shows random distributions of cells.

Disadvantage

It is a difficult method to learn and perform. Also the cover slip gets easily broken.

Centrifugal Method

With the help of centrifuge, a small volume of blood is spun from a central point creating an evenly dispersed monolayer of cells across the slide by the virtue of high torque and low inertia of motion. It is the best method because a single layer of evenly distributed and less distorted cells is obtained.

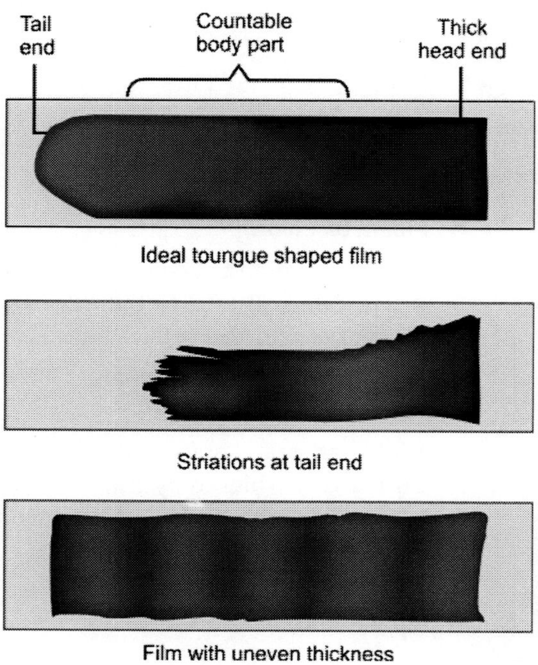

Fig. 7.2: Different types of blood films *(For color version see Plate 4)*

STAINING OF PERIPHERAL SMEAR

A well-stained blood smear is a simple and good tool to study cellular components of blood. An evenly spread thin blood film shows blood cells in single layer. Each cell then can be identified by its characteristic granules and stain properties

Apparatus

1. 4-5 ideal blood smears
2. Staining rack
3. Dropper/Dropping bottle
4. Buffered water (pH-6.8) – At this, pH, stain particles will get ionized and it is in the ionized state only that they can enter the cells and bind to their respective targets. It gives best differential staining.
5. Leishman stain – Commonly used stains are Romanowsky stains. These are prepared by dissolving basic dyes/ thiazines, i.e. methylene blue; and acidic dye, i.e. Eosin, Azure A, B, C in methanol. Depending upon precise proportion of dyes, these stains are given names like Leishman stain, Geimsa stain etc. We use Leishman stain here for staining peripheral blood films. It contains eosin and methylene blue dissolved in acetone and water-free methyl alcohol.
   - *Eosin:* Acidic dye stains basic particles. Eosin reacts with and imparts reddish coloration to basic components of the cell, e.g.
     - Several cytoplasmic components
     - Granules of eosinophils.
     - Hemoglobin
   - Methylene blue: Basic dye stains acidic granules in cytoplasm. Methylene blue

and azures impart blue color to the acid components of the cell like:

- Nucleic acids
- Nuclear proteins
- Heparin containing granules of basophils

Acetone and Water Free Methyl Alcohol

Methyl alcohol serves 2 functions.

- Methyl alcohol precipitates the plasma proteins thus fixing the blood cells to the slide so that they are not washed away during staining.
- It also preserves morphology and chemical status of cells.
- It should be acetone-free because acetone is a strong lipid solvent and if present it will cause crenation, shrinkage or even destruction of cell membrane which will make cell identification difficult. Also presence of acetone will lead to quick deterioration of stain.
- It should be water-free because water if present will lead to rouleaux formation, hemolysis and precipitation of the stain components.

Principle of Staining Procedure

Staining method for blood films fixes dead cells (as opposed to supra vital staining which is used for living cells) and stains cytoplasm and nuclei of cells.

Procedure

Includes fixing and staining.

Fixing the Smear

1. Take 4-5 ideal blood smears.
2. Place the slides; smear side up on a staining rack assembly over a sink (2 metal rods placed across the sink with the ends fitted into short pieces of rubber tubing can also serve the purpose). Ensure that they are horizontal.
3. Pour 8-10 drops of Leishman stain (with a dropper/dropping bottles containing stain) on each slide enough to cover the smear. It should not run off.
4. Note the time. Leave it for about 2 minutes. This is the fixation time when methyl alcohol precipitates proteins of the smear. No staining occurs during this time as the stain particles are in non-ionized form and cannot enter cells.
5. Watch the stain carefully. During hot weather, stain may become syrupy (thick) due to evaporation of alcohol. If stain dries it will precipitate on blood film and appear as round blue granules when examined under microscope. Adding more stain on the slide when it starts becoming thick can prevent this.

Staining the Smear

1. At the end of fixation, add equal number of drops (8-10) of buffered water (pH 6.8) over the smear with a dropper.
2. Water should not spill over.
3. Mix stain and buffered water evenly by gently blowing air intermittently.
4. The smear will have a glossy greenish layer (scum) on its surface.
5. Allow the stain to remain on the slide for 8-10 minutes (Staining time).
6. Flush off the diluted stain in a gentle stream of distilled water, with the slide in the slanting position for about 30 sec-2 min. The film gets a pinkish tinge. None of the greenish scum should settle on the surface of the film. Water should not strike the blood film directly otherwise the film can be washed off.
7. Dry the slides by waving in air.

Precautions

1. Smear should be completely dry before staining otherwise it will get removed on washing.
2. Staining should be done within 2 hours of smear preparation
3. Put adequate amount of stain so that it covers the whole smear. Give adequate fixing time.
4. Don't let the stain to go dry on the smear, if required add more drops of stain to prevent drying else it will lead to deposition of stain particles.
5. Use freshly prepared, adequately filtered stain to avoid deposition of stain particles on the smear.
6. Fix, stain and wash the smear for adequate time. Under fixing, under staining or over washing can give faded/red (if stain is more acidic) appearance.
7. Over fixing, over staining or under washing can give the stain excessively blue appearance.

EXAMINATION OF STAINED SAMER

Assessment of Stained Blood Smear

Examine the smear with naked eye first. Check the staining and thickness of the blood smear by examining it under low power and then under high power objective.

Features of a Well-stained Blood Smear

Naked Eye Appearance

Smear appears translucent, and bluish pink when seen against a white surface; thickness is uniform throughout.

Under Low Power (10x)

Smear is one cell thick, without overlapping of cells. Cells are uniformly distributed where in red cells appear as dots, and WBC cannot be differentiated.

Under High Power (40x)

Red cells are stained orange buff or pink. WBCs are stained with their nuclei deep blue violet.

Examination of Stained Smear Under Oil Immersion

1. Place a small drop of cedarwood oil in the center of smear. Swing the oil immersion objective into position. Carefully lower the objective till it just touches the oil drop.
2. Focus the cells using fine adjustment.
3. Study the distribution of different types of cells throughout the length of the smear.

Identification of Cells

The most abundant cells seen are RBCs, which appears light pinkish, non-nucleated and disc shaped.

The WBCs, which are nucleated, are lesser in number and larger than red cells. Observe the following characteristic features to identify the various leukocytes.

GRANULES

Presence or Absence of granules,

Size: Granules can be Large and coarse (pinhead sized) or Small and fine (pin point sized).

Color: Color of granules can be deep blue black, neutral or brick red.

SIZE OF THE CELL

Size is determined by comparing WBCs with surrounding red cells (7.2 - 7.8 μm). WBC size can be:

- Similar to the size of RBCs
- Double the size of RBCs
- Triple the size of RBCs

IDENTIFICATION OF LEUKOCYTES

Table 7.1: Types of leukocytes

Type of leukocyte	*Size as compared to RBCs*	*Nucleus*	*Granules*	*Cytoplasm*	*Nucleus to cytoplasm ratio*
Neutrophil	Double (10-14 μm)	• Stained blue • Multi-lobed, lobes joined by thin chromatin filament	• Present • Fine (pin point sized) • Pinkish, • Numerous and uniformly scattered through out cytoplasm	Faintly lilac stained	
Eosinophil	Double (10-14 μm)	• Stained blue in contrast to red granules • Bilobed connected by thick chromatin strand (Spectacle appearance)	• Present • Coarse (pin head sized) • Round • Brick red to orange granules • May obscure nucleus	Light pink containing granules	
Large lymphocyte	Double (10-14 μm)	• Violet in color • Oval or rounded, with or without a dent • Compact and homogeneous	• Absent	Clear, light blue color	80 : 20 Nucleus occupies 80-90% of cell volume
Small lymphocyte	Same (7-8 μm)	• Deep violet in color Homogeneous (Ink drop appearance)	• Absent	Clear blue, thin rim of cytoplasm, present at periphery	90 : 10 Nucleus occupies almost whole cell
Monocycte	Triple (12-24 μm) Largest WBC	Heterogeneous Staining • Spongy appearance • Eccentric • Kidney/horse shoe/rounded or dumbbell shaped	• Absent, • Very occasionally red stained rod like **Auer body/granules** are present in 15% monocytes. They are always few in contrast to granules	Hazy ground glass in appearance • May show presence of vacuoles	50 : 50 Nucleus occupies 50% of cell volume
Basophil	Double (10-14 μm)	• Bilobed or • Trilobed • Studded with granules	• Present • Blue black • Coarse, fills cells and obscure nucleus and cell boundary	Obscured by granules	

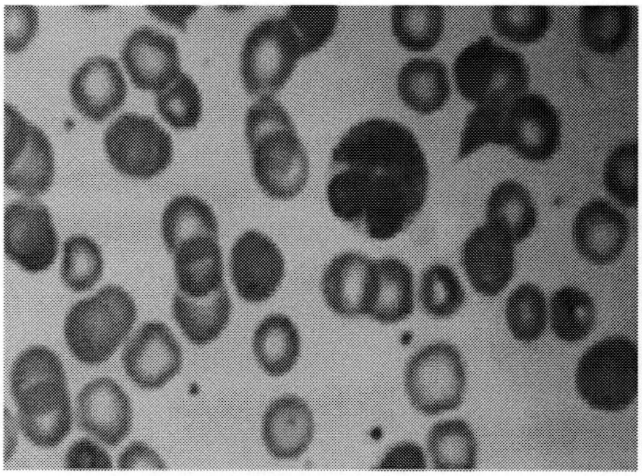

Eosinophil
(For color version see Plate 5)

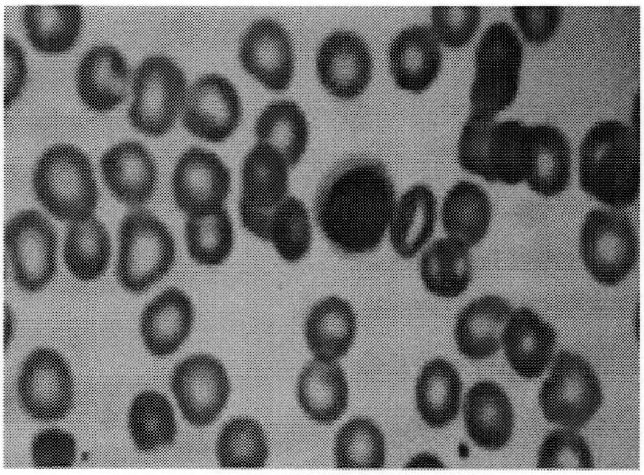

Large lymphocyte
(For color version see Plate 5)

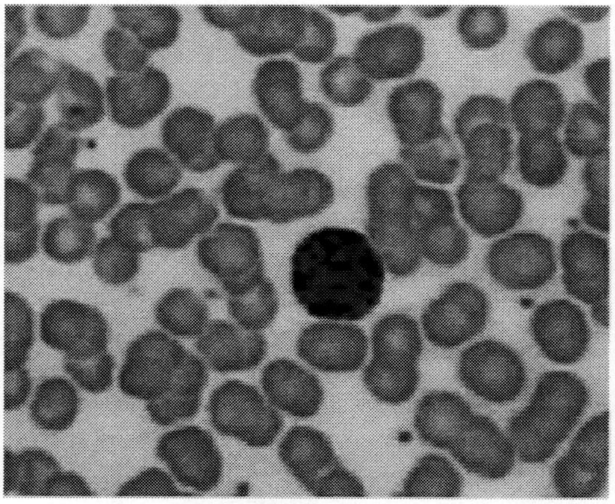

Basophil
(For color version see Plate 5)

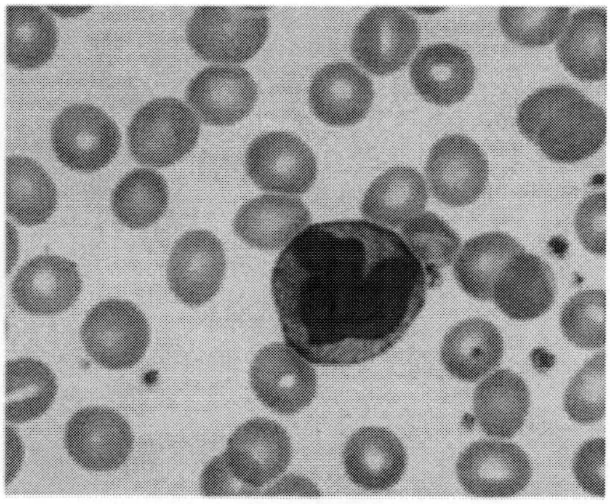

Monocyte
(For color version see Plate 5)

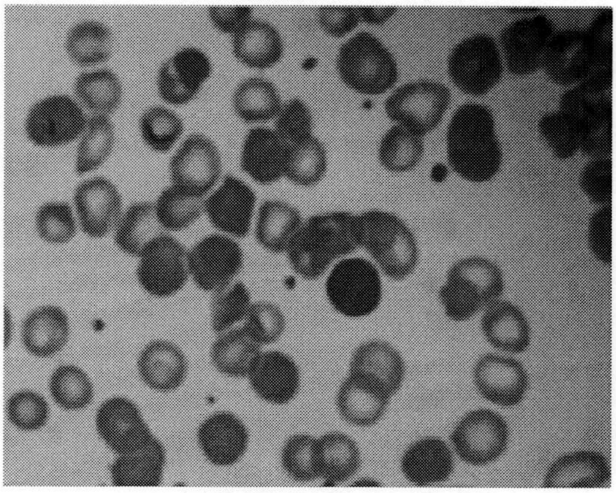

Small lymphocyte
(For color version see Plate 5)

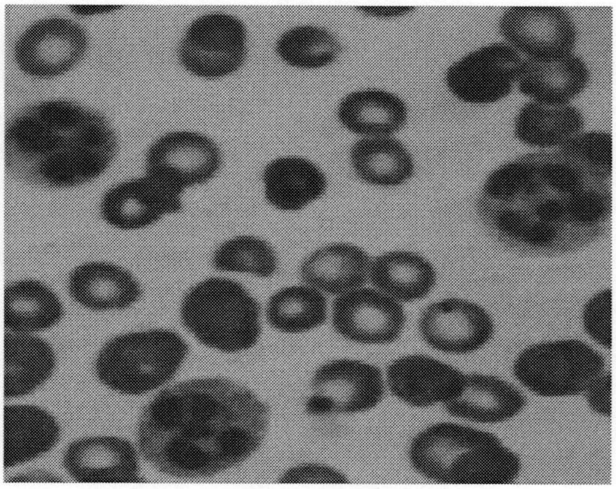

Neutrophil
(For color version see Plate 5)

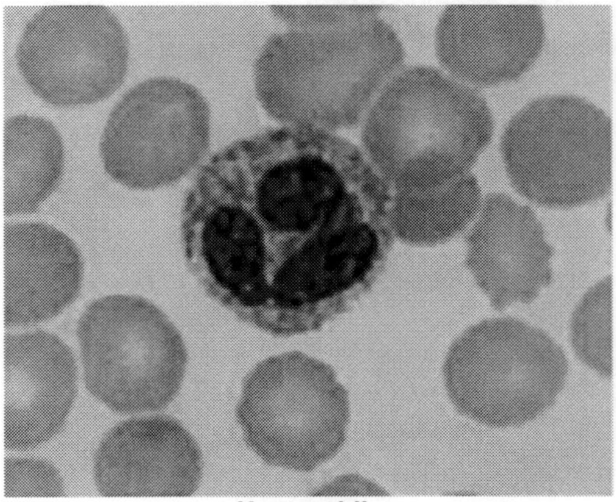

Neutrophil
(For color version see Plate 6)

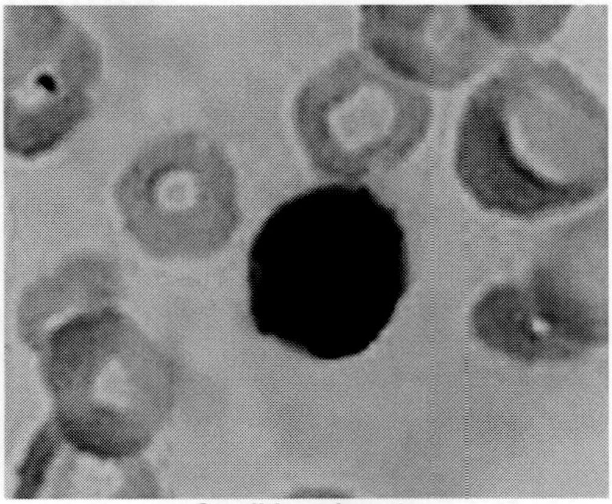

Small lymphocyte
(For color version see Plate 6)

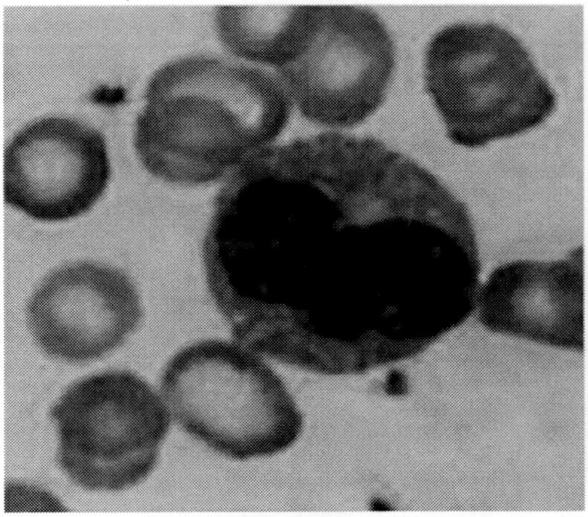

Monocyte
(For color version see Plate 6)

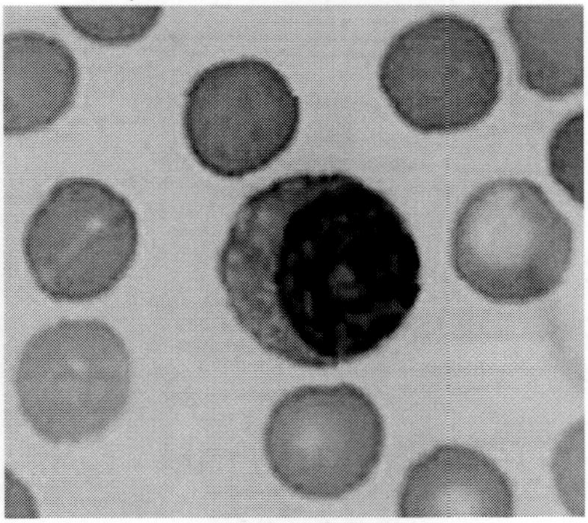

Large lymphocyte
(For color version see Plate 6)

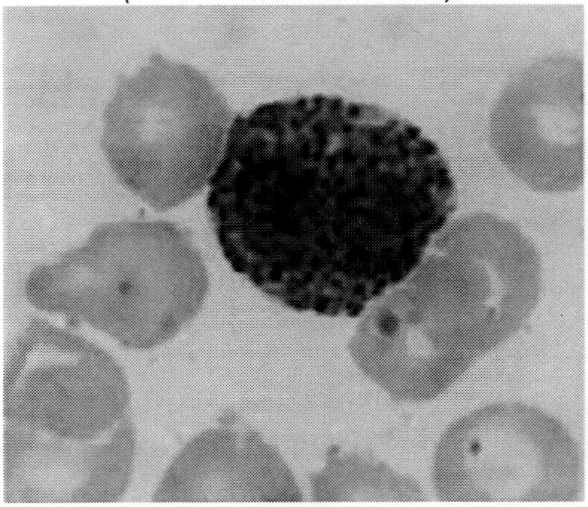

Basophil
(For color version see Plate 6)

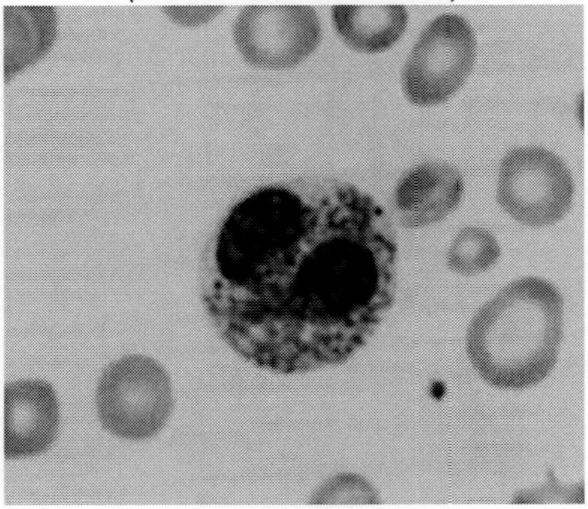

Eosinophil
(For color version see Plate 6)

NUCLEUS

Its color, shapes and lobes are to be noted
Color: Pink or purple
Shape: Round, oval, horse shoe/ kidney
Location: Central, eccentric

Lobes

Number of lobes
Thickness of chromatin, attaching the lobes.
Chromatin: Condensed or open and reticular.

CYTOPLASM

Color: Light violet or pink
Staining pattern: Homogeneous or heterogeneous.

CYTOPLASM TO NUCLEUS RATIO

Note amount of cytoplasm in relation to size of cell and nucleus.

DISCUSSION

Over/Under Staining

If smear is over stained, i.e. it has totally purple appearance and the red cells appear bluish black. Nuclei of WBC are stained dark blue and there is bluish cytoplasm in all cells then wash the slide under running water for 1-2 min.

If it is under stained, i.e. red cells appear pale pink and WBCs are almost colorless, it can be restained

Distribution of Cells in the Smear

At the head-end of smear:

- RBCs are crowded and superimposed
- WBCs are poorly stained.

At the tail end of smear:

- Cells are wide apart
- WBCs are distorted
- Neutrophils, monocytes predominate at the margins and tail end (dragged there by spreader because of their large size).

At the upper and lower edges of smear:

- WBCs are plenty, poorly stained, and abnormally rich in granules.

In the body (the middle part) of the smear:

- Lymphocytes are abundant.
- Body of the smear should be used for counting cells.

WORK SPACE

ANSWER THESE QUESTIONS

Q1. Draw different types of WBCs seen under microscope.

Large lymphocyte	Monocyte

Small lymphocyte	Neutrophil
Eosinophil	**Basophil**

Q2. Differentiate between a Neutrophil and an Eosinophil.

Characters	Neutrophil	Eosinophil

Q3. Differentiate between Large Lymphocyte from a Monocyte.

Characters	Large Lymphocyte	Monocyte

Q4. What is the composition of Leishman stain? What are the functions of its each component?

VIVA QUESTIONS

Q1. What precautions are taken for preparing a blood smear?
Q2. Which factors determine the smear thickness?
Q3. Why smear should always be dried quickly soon after spreading it?
Q4. What are the features of an ideal smear?
Q5. Why water is not used as solvent for Leishman stain?
Q6. Why should the methyle alcohal be acetone and water-free?
Q7. Why Leishman stain is diluted after 1-2 minutes not earlier?
Q8. Why the cells don't get stained during first two minutes (fixing time) of staining procedure?
Q9. Why buffered water is preferred over distilled or tap water?
Q10. What is the significance of appearance of scum on the staining fluid after addition of water?

CHAPTER

8

Determination of Differential Leukocyte Count

OBJECTIVE

After completing the practical student should:

- Know different methods of counting different leukocytes
- Know importance of performing DLC
- Be able to perform DLC
- Know the reasons for neutrophila, neutropenia, eosinophilia, eosinopenia, basophilia, basopenia, monocytosis and monocytopenia
- Know the normal percentage of each leukocyte.

INTRODUCTION

Determination of percentage distribution of leukocytes in peripheral blood is known as Differential Leukocyte Count.

Principle

A stained blood film is examined under oil immersion objective and different types of cells are identified. The percentage distribution of the cells is then determined.

Apparatus

1. A well stained smear
2. Microscope
3. Cedarwood oil

Procedure

1. Take the best-stained slide.
2. Put a drop of cedarwood oil on it and focus under oil immersion lens.
3. Start from one end of the smear. Identify the leukocyte that you come across, count it and enter it in your observation record.
4. For counting cells, bring one corner, say left upper corner of the film in view. Shift slide towards the left along the same horizontal axis to bring adjacent field in view. Traverse through out the length of the film. Then move slide vertically by a distance equivalent to 2 mm and again traverse full length of film in opposite direction. Then again shift lower down and go on counting towards left again and so on (As showing in Fig. 8.1).
5. Complete the count of cells in whole film in this zigzag manner. Enter your observations using any one of the method described below.
   I. By using counting machine which has different keys for different types of cells. Pressing any key records and adds the number.

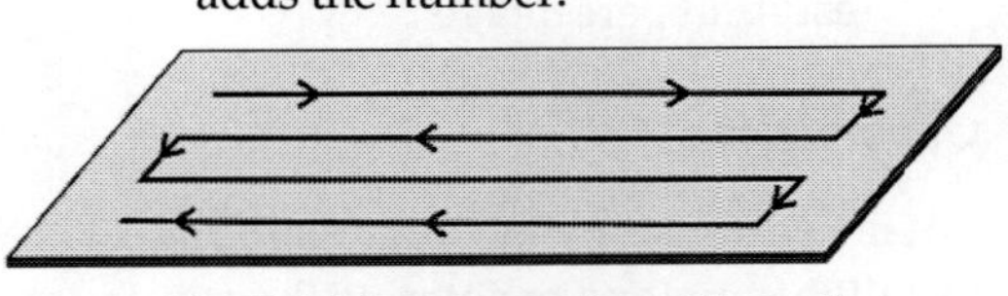

Fig. 8.1: Zigzag way of counting cells

II. Tally bar method of counting cells – Prepare columns for identifying each type of cell and label them. Each cell identified is denoted by making a small vertical line (of the same type under one column) and fifth cell counted is represented with a diagonal line crossing the first four lines.

NEUTROPHILS	𝍸 𝍸 𝍸 𝍸 𝍸 𝍸 𝍸 𝍸	= 40
MONOCYTES	𝍸 III	= 8
BASOPHILS	I	= 1
LYMPHOCYTE	𝍸 𝍸 𝍸 𝍸	= 20
EOSINOPHILS	𝍸 𝍸 II	= 12

III. Mark out adequate number of squares (not less than 100) on a piece of paper. After identifying each cell it is entered by writing a letter say N for neutrophil, E for eosinophil and so on.

N	N	N	N	N	N	N	M	N	N
L	L	N	N	N	N	L	SL	L	L
SL	L	N	SL	N	L	N	L	N	M
N	N	N	N	N	L	E	N	E	M
N	N	N	N	N	L	L	SL	N	N
L	N	N	N	N	L	N	SL	N	M
SL	N	N	N	M	N	L	SL	N	N
M	E	N	N	N	N	N	L	L	L
L	N	N	N	M	M	N	L	N	L
L	L	N	E	N	L	L	L	L	L

6. Count minimum of 100 cells and give the results in percentage.

Observations

Enter your observation after counting 100 cells by tallybar method or entering them in squares.

Precautions

1. For DLC the film should be prepared from a small but a whole drop of freely flowing blood. Otherwise the count obtained may not represent the true blood picture.
2. Count cells through out the length of the smear except extreme ends of head and tail.
3. Counting should be done in zigzag manner to prevent double counting of cells. Body or middle part of smear should be used for counting cells.
4. Minimum of 100 cells should be counted

Result

Express your result as
N – Neutrophil = 54%
E – Eosinophil = 4%
B – Basophil = 0%
M – Monocyte = 8%
L – Lymphocyte (SNL-small and L-large) = 34%

Normal Differential Leukocyte Count

Neutrophils: 50-70%
Eosinophils: 1-4%
Basophils: 0-1%
Monocytes: 2-8%
Lymphocyte: 20-40%

Discussion

For DLC if the drop of the blood is small count all the cells of the film but if drop is large counting has to be restricted. The approximate number of cells to be counted depends upon the TLC, e.g.

Table 8.1: Approximate number of cells to be counted for DLC

TLC	*Minimum No. of cells to be counted for DLC*
5000	100
10000	200
20000	300
Above 20000	400

Absolute leukocyte count can also be calculated by using the value of TLC along with DLC to express the percentage in terms of absolute values of each type of leukocyte per mm^3 of blood. Absolute values are more significant than DLC values alone.

Table 8.2: Absolute leukocyte count

Type of leukocytes	*Percentage obtained*	*Cells per mm^3*
Neutrophils	40-75	2000-7500
Eosinophils	1-6	4-440
Basophils	0-1	0 - 100
Monocytes	2-10	500-800
Lymphocyte	20-45	1300-3500

DLC along with TLC is also used to detect infection/inflammation, to determine the efficiency of drugs, chemotherapy, radiation, etc. to monitor blood diseases: leukemia, to detect allergic and parasitic infections

CONDITIONS WHICH ALTERS DLC

Neutrophilia: Increase in the neutrophil count

Physiological Causes

I. Exercise
II. Pregnancy
III. After meals
IV. Emotional stress
V. Cold exposure

Pathological Causes

I. Acute pyogenic infections
II. All bacterial infections except typhoid fever
III. Myocardial infarction
IV. Acute hemorrhage
V. Burns, tissue trauma

Neutropenia: Decrease in the neutrophil count

Physiological Causes

I. In children

Pathological Causes

I. Typhoid fever, paratyphoid
II. Viral infections – measles, hepatitis and influenza
III. Bone marrow depression
IV. Aplastic anemia

Eosinophilia: Increase in eosinophil count

I. Allergic conditions like
 - Bronchial asthma
 - Urticaria
 - Hay fever

II. Parasitic infestations
 - Hookworm
 - Filariasis

III. Skin diseases
 - Pemphigus
 - Psoriasis

Eosinopenia: Decrease in eosinophil count

I. ACTH therapy
II. Cushing's disease
III. Aplastic anemia

Basophilia: Increase in basophil count

I. Chronic myeloid leukemia
II. Viral infections
III. Allergic diseases
IV. Smallpox
V. Chicken pox

Basopenia: Decrease in basophil count

I. Severe septicemia
II. Aplastic anemia
III. Glucocorticoid therapy

Monocytosis: Increase in monocytes count

I. Malaria
II. Infectious mononucleosis
III. Kala azar

IV. Subacute bacterial endocarditic

V. Hodgkin's disease

VI. ACTH therapy

Monocytopenia: Decrease in monocyte count

I. Bone marrow failure

II. Aplastic anemia

III. Septicemia

Lymphocytosis: Increase in lymphocyte count

I. Relative lymphocytosis in children

II. Chronic infections

III. Tuberculosis

IV. Syphilis

V. Lymphoma

VI. Viral infection

Lymphopenia: Decrease in lymphocyte count

I. Immunosuppressive therapy

II. ACTH therapy

III. AIDS

IV. Bone marrow failure

WORK SPACE

Name Age Sex

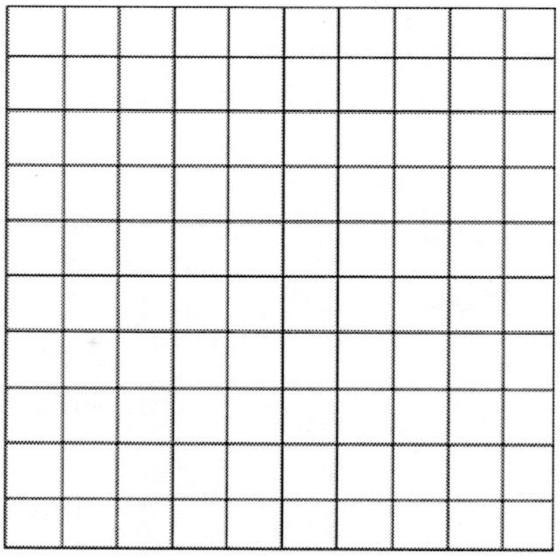

Result

Inference

ANSWER THESE QUESTIONS

Q1. Enumerate different functions of neutrophils, eosinophils, lymphocytes and monocytes.

Q2. Which part of the blood film should be used for counting cells?

VIVA QUESTIONS

Q1. What is the normal percentage distribution of various leucocytes?
Q2. Why it is important to study the whole length of the smear?
Q3. What is the significance of performing DLC?
Q4. What are the conditions where neutrophilia is seen?
Q5. What are the conditions where neutropenia is seen?
Q6. What are the conditions where eosinophilia is seen?
Q7. What are the conditions where eosinopenia is seen?
Q8. What are the conditions where bosopenia is seen?
Q9. What are the conditions where bosophilia is seen?
Q10. What are the conditions where monocytopenia is seen?
Q11. What are the conditions where monocytosis is seen?
Q12. What are the conditions where lymphocytosis is seen?
Q13. What are the conditions where lymphocytopenia is seen?

CHAPTER 9

Determination of Hemoglobin Concentration in Blood

OBJECTIVES

After completing the practical student should:

- Be able to enumerate different methods for estimation of hemoglobin (Hb).
- Be able to estimate Hb by Sahli's method
- Know the principle of Sahli's method
- Know the precautions observed
- Know which method is best for Hb estimation
- Know advantages and disadvantages of sahli's method
- Be aware of physiological and pathological variations of Hb concentration
- Know normal values of Hb concentration in adult males and females.
- Know different types and derivatives of Hb.

INTRODUCTION

Hemoglobin (Hb) concentration is almost always determined as part of routine laboratory investigation. It is indicated in all disorders of blood (like anemias leukemias), chronic diseases, tuberculosis, malignancies, renal failure and before all surgical operations.

Methods

Hemoglobinometery is the method of determining amount of hemoglobin in blood. There are different methods of measuring Hb concentration. Most frequently employed method for routine Hb estimation is Sahli's method.

Sahli's Method for Determination of Hb

Principle: The amount of hemoglobin is estimated by conversion of a known volume of blood to acid hematin by addition with N/10 HCl and comparing with a suitable standard. Blood on dilution with HCl turns golden brown in color. The intensity of the color depends upon concentration of acid hematin which in turn depends on concentration of Hb. The color of the solution after dilution with water is matched against golden brown tinted glass rods by direct vision. The readings are obtained in gm%.

Apparatus

1. Material for sterile finger prick
2. Dropper
3. N/10 or (0.1N) HCl –
   - It will hemolyze RBCs and convert Hb into acid hematin.
   - Only N/10 HCl can be used in Sahli's method because this method is standardized for N/10 HCl and any strong acid or alkali (strong oxidizing agent) if used in its place they will damage Hb proteins thus interfering in its estimation.
4. Distilled water
   - It is used for diluting the acid hematin formed so as to match its color with standard glass rods.

- It is preferred over tap water because salts in tap water will lead to turbidity and interfere with color matching.
- N/10 HCl can be used for dilution because it doesn't cause turbidity and effect the color of the solution (all the Hb has already been converted into acid hematin, N/10 cannot further effect the color of the solution) but being costlier than distilled water it is not used.

5. Sahli's hemoglobinometer – It includes:
   - *Comparator:* It is a rectangular plastic box with a slot in the middle to accommodate the calibrated Hb tube. Non-fading standardized golden brown glass rods are fitted on each side of the slot. The opaque white background provides the necessary contrast and illumination for direct visual color matching and easy comparison.
   - *Hb Pipette:* It is without any bulb and has only one mark indicating 20 mm^3 (0.02 ml)
   - *Hb tube:* round/square tube graduated from 20-140 percentage on one side and 2-24 gm% on other side. Of the 2 scales given on the Hb tubes, the g% scale is used, because that is what is required. The scale in % is of no value; except for academic interest. There is not a single standard value of hemoglobin which is taken as 100%.
   - *Stirrer:* It is a thin glass rod with a flat end used for mixing blood and acid in the Hb tube.

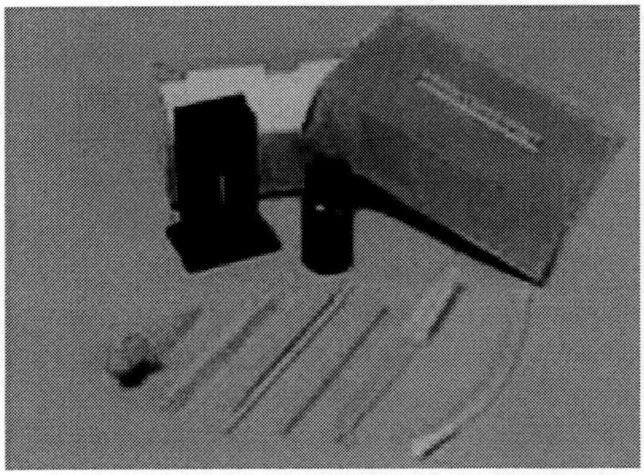

Fig. 9.1: Hemoglobinometer

Procedure

1. With the help of a dropper, fill the Hb tube with N/10 HCl upto the lowest mark (upto mark 20% or 2 gm%) and set it aside.
2. Prick the finger under aseptic conditions; wipe away the first drop of blood. Let a large drop of free-flowing blood form.
3. Draw blood exactly upto 20 mm^3 mark into the Hb pipette; taking care, there should not be any air bubble (if any air bubble enters discard the pipette and take a new one).
4. Wipe off any blood from the outside of the tip. Avoid touching the bore/else blood will be drawn out by capillary action.
5. Immediately immerse the tip of the pipette to the bottom of the acid solution in Hb tube and expel the blood gently.
6. Rinse the pipette 3-4 times by drawing up and blowing out the acid solution till all blood is washed out from the pipette. Avoid foaming/frothing of mixture.
7. Withdraw the pipette from the tube, without touching it to the side of the tube, thus ensuring no mixture is carried out of the tube.
8. Using the flat end of the stirrer mix the blood with the acid solution.
9. Put the Hb tube in the comparator and let it stand for 10 min. During this time acid ruptures the red cells, release the Hb and converts Hb to acid hematin giving deep golden brown color to the solution.

10. After 10 min add a drop of distilled water to the solution and mix it.
11. After adding 2-3 drops of distilled water and mixing compare the color with the standard glass rods of the comparator
12. For comparing the color:
    - Hold the comparator at the arms length and at the level of eyes and against the sun light (indirect diffuse but bright light)
    - Lift the stirrer above the solution only and not out of the tube
    - Turn the tube to avoid viewing through the markings on it.
13. Continue dilution till solution color matches that of the standard. Note the reading of the lower meniscus.

OBSERVATIONS

Take three readings.

First: When color of solution is slightly darker than standard.

Second: When it matches the standard.

Third: When it becomes slightly lighter than standard.

RESULT

Take the average of 3 readings and express your result as:

Hemoglobin concentration

= .... gm/100 ml blood

Precautions

1. Accurate amount of N/10 HCl should be taken in Hb tube.
    - If less N/10 HCl is added blood may clot or all Hb will not be converted into acid hematin
    - If more N/10 HCl is added final color developed will be very light (especially in case of anemia) it will be impossible to match the color because solution can't be concentrated.
2. All precautions mentioned for collecting capillary blood must be observed.
3. Wipe off any blood from the outside of the tip with non-absorbent material.
4. Avoid touching the bore with absorbent material else blood will be drawn out by capillary action.
5. Blood should be transferred quickly to tube containing N/10 HCl to prevent clotting of blood in pipette.
6. Frothing should not occur when blood is expelled in the Hb tube. There shouldn't be any air bubble in the Hb tube.
7. Blood should be allowed to be acted upon by acid for at least 10 min. The color of acid hematin does not develop fully immediately but its intensity increase with time reaching a maximum, after which it starts decreasing.
    - Too little time: All Hb may not be converted to acid hematin
    - Too long time: Result in fading of color.

    In either case, result will be falsely a low.
8. While comparing the color, stirrer should be lifted above the solution. If stirrer is left in the solution, solution will appear light.
9. At no stage the stirrer should be completely taken out of the tube. It will lead to loss of solution.
10. Distilled water should be added drop by drop to avoid over dilution.
11. While matching color, solution should be golden brown throughout the solution. Dark color at the bottom indicates poor mixing.
12. Matching of colors should be done against natural sources of light.
13. While matching, keep the Hb tube in a way so that the calibrations should not interfere in the color matching.
14. Read the lower meniscus for the Hb value.
15. Three readings should be taken to reduce personal error.

Advantages of Sahli's Method

1. Simple, does not require costly equipment.
2. Only requires direct visual color matching.
3. Fairly quick and accurate.
4. Can be used in mass surveys for anemias.

Disadvantages of Sahli's Method

1. Since acid hematin is not a true solution, some turbidity may occur.
2. The method estimates only oxyHb and reduced Hb. Other forms of Hb like carboxyHb, metHb and sulfHb are not estimated.
3. Also the degree of error could be quite high if suitable precautions are not taken.
4. The color of the standard glass rods may fade with time.

Sources of Errors

Giving False High Value

1. Blood taken more than 20 mm^3.
2. Blood sticking outside the pipette tip.
3. Fading of standard colored glass rods.

Giving False Low Value

1. Blood sample diluted with tissue fluid
2. Blood sample less than 20 mm^3.
3. If N/10 HCl is added less than required amount, less hemoglobin will be converted into acid hematin.
4. Color of acid hematin not allowed to develop fully.

NORMAL VALUES

Males: 14 - 18 g/dl
Females: 12- 16 g/dl
New borns: 16-22 gm/dl

DISCUSSION

Functions of Hemoglobin

Hemoglobin is a pigment present in red cells. It gives red color to blood. Its synthesis requires iron, proteins, copper, nickel, cobalt, pyridoxine, riboflavin, nicotinic acid, Vit C, etc. It has many functions in body:

- Carries O_2 from lungs to all tissues
- Carries CO_2 from tissues to lungs
- Hb acts as buffer. 75% of buffering power of blood is because of Hb
- Hemoglobin interacts with nitric oxide (NO) to regulate the blood pressure. The interaction of NO with hemoglobin leads to the formation of S-nitrosothiols or SNO. In the lungs where oxygenated blood is present, the release of CO_2 from the hemoglobin and its oxygenation are associated with formation of SNO. Oxygen release in the tissues is associated with SNO release also. Native hemoglobin leads to the elevation of blood pressure but the SNO-hemoglobin do not exert the same effect. Therefore, the function of hemoglobin does not seem to be merely confined to its vital role of tissue oxygenation, rather this molecule actively participates in the regulation of blood pressure.

Derivatives of Hemoglobin

There are different Hb derivatives like—

- OxyHb: When Hb combines with O_2
- Reduced Hb: When O_2 is released from oxyHb
- Carboxy Hb: Hb combines with CO
- Carbamino Hb: Hb combines with CO_2
- MetHb: When ferrous of Hb is converted into ferric ion, due to exposure to certain drugs or oxidizing agents it forms Met Hb

- CyanmetHb: Formed by the action of cyanide on Hb
- SulfHb: Formed by the action of certain drugs like sulphonamides on Hb.

Varieties of Hb

Each molecule of Hb has 4 subunits. Each subunit consists of heme conjugated to a polypeptide chain depending on the type of polypeptide chains present, there are different types of Hb, e.g.

Hb A

- It has two α (alpha) chains and two β (beta) chains
- It is adult Hb
- About 95% of Hb present in normal adult is Hb A.

HbA$_2$

- It has two α chains and two δ (delta) chains
- About 5% of Hb present in normal adult is Hb A$_2$.

Hb F

- It has two α chains and two γ (gamma) chains
- It is fetal Hb
- At birth, fetal hemoglobin comprises about 75-95% of the child's hemoglobin. These levels decline after six months when adult hemoglobin synthesis is activated while fetal hemoglobin synthesis is deactivated
- The γ subunit of fetal hemoglobin has less affinity for 2, 3-bisphosphoglycerate as compared to adult hemoglobin (2, 3-BPG lowers the Hb affinity for O_2). This means that fetal hemoglobin has more affinity to O_2 and the maternal adult hemoglobin has less O_2 affinity. So the hemoglobin of the mother readily transfers its oxygen to the fetal hemoglobin
- Fetal hemoglobin's affinity for oxygen is substantially greater than that of adult hemoglobin. Notably, the P50 value for fetal hemoglobin (i.e. the partial pressure of oxygen at which the Hb is 50% saturated; lower values indicate greater affinity) is roughly 19 mm Hg, whereas adult hemoglobin has a value of approximately 26.8 mm Hg. As a result, the oxygen saturation curve, is left-shifted for fetal hemoglobin in comparison to the same curve in adult hemoglobin
- Fetal Hb is also more resistant to action of alkalies and its this property is utilized for its estimation.

Other Fetal Hemoglobins

Bart's Hb

- Minor Hb presnt in fetal life
- Contains four γ chains
- Its concentration increases in fetal life in thalassemia.

Gower 1

- It has two ζ (zeta)chains and two ξ (epsilon) chains.

Gower 2

- It has two α chains and two ξ (epsilon) chains.

Portland

- It has two ζ (zeta)chains and two γ chains.

Thalassemia

It's a genetic defect where either α or β chain is absent (major thalassemia) or less in amount (minor thalassemia) resulting in anemia.

Hemoglobinopathies

It includes conditions where abnormal Hb chains are formed, e.g.

HbS

- It has normal α chains but in β chain one glutamic acid residue is replaced by valine residue
- Its presence lead to sickle cell anemia
- Under low oxygen tension HbS crystallizes and cells become sickle shaped.

HbC

- It has normal α chains but in β chain glutamic acid residue at 6th position is replaced by lysine residue.

HEMOGLOBINOMETERY

It refers to measurement of concentration of Hb in blood. There are different methods of Hb estimation.

1. Gasometric Method

It is based on oxygen carrying capacity of Hb. A sample of blood is exposed to pure O_2. Hb gets saturated with O_2 and the amount of O_2 is then determined by using van Slyke apparatus. Since, 1 gm of Hb combines with 1.34 ml of O_2, knowing the O_2 carrying capacity gives the amount of Hb in that sample. Though it is an accurate method but complicated for routine work.

2. Estimate of Iron Content

Iron in blood is separated with sulphuric acid and its amount is measured. Since 1 gm of Hb contains 3.35 mg of iron, estimating the iron concentration can indirectly indicate the Hb concentration.

3. Tallquist's Method

A drop of blood is absorbed on a white filter paper and allowed to spread to form an even spot. As soon as the spot loses its shine and before it dries it is matched against a scale of increasingly dark red colored round spots printed on a card representing various concentration of hemoglobin expressed in %.

4. Copper Sulphate Falling Drop Method

It is a rapid method for estimating approximate level of Hb and it is used in large surveys. It compares the specific gravity of blood with specific gravity of a series of copper sulphate solutions. Line charts/tables are consulted to read off the concentration values.

5. Spectrophotometric method/photoelectric colorimetry

When light is passed through a solution of oxyHb or reduced Hb specific wavelength of light is absorbed. By using a photo-electric colorimeter the amount of light absorbed by the solution is measured. The light used in colorimeter is of limited wave band and this wave band is chosen to correspond with the part of spectrum that is maximally absorbed by the solution being tested.

I. *Cyanmethemoglobin method/Drabkins method:* This method is most accurate for routine estimation of Hb estimation because it estimates all forms of Hb (oxyHb, reducedHb, carboxyHb and metHb). The blood sample is treated with modified Drabkin's reagent which is a solution of potassium cyanide, potassium ferricy-anide and potassium phosphate. All forms of Hb are converted into a single stable compound – cyanmetHb. The amount of light absorbed with yellow green filters

(540 mm wavelength) is compared with a standard solution of cyanmethemoglobin.

II. *Haldane's carboxyhemoglobin method:* Red cells are hemolyzed in distilled water to release Hb and carbon monoxide is passed through the solution to form carboxyHb which is bright red in color. Its color is compared with a standard solution.

III. *Oxyhemoglobin method:* Hb is fully oxygenated by treating blood with sodium carbonate/ammonium hydroxide and the solution is compared with a standard grey screen in a colorimeter.

IV. *Wu's alkaline hematin method:* Blood is treated with N/10 NaOH which converts all forms of Hb to alkaline hematin and then compared with the standard at 540 mm. It doesn't estimate HbF content in the blood.

Causes of Increase in Hemoglobin Concentration

Physiological

- In males due to testosterone hormone
- In newborns due to intrauterine hypoxic conditions
- At high altitude due to hypoxia.

Pathological

- Polycythemia rubra Vera
- Chronic hypoxia
- Cardiorespiratory disorders.

Causes of Decrease in Hemoglobin Concentration

Physiological

- In females because of presence of estrogen which is inhibitory to erythropoiesis
- During pregnancy due to hemodilution.

Pathological

All causes of anemia.

WORK SPACE

Name Age Sex

Observations

Readings	*Color compared to glass rods*	*Value in gm%*
1st	Slightly darker than standard	
2nd	Similar to the standard	
3rd	Slightly lighter than standard	

Calculation

Result

Inference

ANSWER THESE QUESTIONS

Q1. What are the different methods of Hb estimation?

Q2. Which routinely done method is most accurate for Hb estimation and why?

Q3. What is the principle of Sahli's method of Hb estimation?

Q4. Give normal value of Hb in adults.

Q5. Why Hb concentration is more in males and less in females?

Q6. Why Hb concentration is more in newborns than in adult?

VIVA QUESTIONS

Q1. Which method is most preferred method for Hb estimation in mass surveys?

Q2. Which method is most frequently employed method for routine Hb estimation?

Q3. What are the advantages and disadvantages of Sahli's method of Hb estimation?

Q4. What precautions should be taken for Hb estimation?

Q5. Why it is important to wait for 10 minutes before adding distilled water?

Q6. Can tap water or any strong acid or alkali be used for dilution in place of distilled water?

Q7. Why it is important to take accurate amount of N/10 HCl?

Q8. Why N/10 HCl if used for dilution will not affect the color of solution?

Q9. What is hemoglobin?

Q10. Name some of the derivatives of Hb.

Q11. Give different varieties of Hb.

Q12. What are the functions of Hb?

CHAPTER

10

Determination of Blood Groups

OBJECTIVES

After completing the practical student should:

- Know different blood group systems
- Be able to describe physiological basic of blood grouping
- Be able to tell indications or uses of blood grouping
- Determine his ABO and Rh blood group
- Know the precautions observed for determining blood group
- Know the prerequisites of blood transfusion
- Know the indications of blood transfusion.

INTRODUCTION

There are more than 30 blood group systems with more than 300 antigens. Clinically, only three blood group systems are important. These are:

1. ABO system
2. Rh system
3. M and N system

Method of Determination of Blood Group

There are two commonly used methods:

1. Slide method
2. Tube method

Slide Method of Blood Group Determination

Principle

The red cells bear different agglutinogens (isoantigens) on their membrane surface which are glycoproteins. Plasma contains agglutinins (antibodies). The red cell antigens are allowed to react with sera containing known antibodies. The presence or absence of agglutination is then detected by naked eye as well as under the microscope indicating blood group of the individual.

Apparatus

1. Microscope
2. Sterile lancet
3. Sterile gauze
4. Methylated spirit
5. Glass-marking pencil
6. Glass slides
7. Dropper
8. 0.9% saline
9. Watch glass
10. Antisera A, B, D. Anti A, Anti B and Anti D can be obtained by injecting the respective antigen into a rabbit and collecting the antibodies formed from their serum.

    Anti A, B can also be obtained from individuals with blood group B or A respectively

Antiserum A: It is blue in color. Contains monoclonal antibodies (against humans) called Anti-A or α agglutinins. Can be obtained from a person with blood group B.

Antiserum B: It is yellow in color. Contains monoclonal antibodies (against humans) called

Anti-B or β agglutinins. Can be obtained from a person with blood group A.

Antiserum D: It is colorless. Contains monoclonal antibodies (against humans) called Anti-Rh (D) antibodies

The antibodies against Rh factor don't occur naturally.

Procedure

1. Take five clean and dry glass slides and a watch glass.
2. With a glass-marking pencil label four slides as expained below:
   - First slide – as A (for antiserum-A).
   - Second slide – as B (for antiserum-B).
   - Third slide – as C (it will act as control; no antiserum will be put on it).
   - Fourth slide – as D (for antiserum-D).
3. Mark each corners of fifth slide as a, b, c and d.
4. Put one drop of antiserum A , B and D on slides marked A, B and D respectively. No antiserum is placed on slide C. It is used as control to avoid false-positive results.
5. Prick the finger under aseptic conditions.
6. Make red cell suspension by adding and mixing two drops of capillary blood to 6-8 drops of 0.9% normal saline taken in a watch glass.
7. Put one drop of red cell suspension on slides A, B, C and D. Red cell suspension is used in place of direct blood drop from finger tip because –
   - Specific agglutinins act best at low temperature and against well diluted cells. With week sera and higher cell concentration, cells may mop up the agglutinins without being agglutinated
   - Dilution of cells allow easy detection of agglutination when present. In undiluted blood red cells form large rouleaux which may be difficult to disperse and mistaken for agglutination

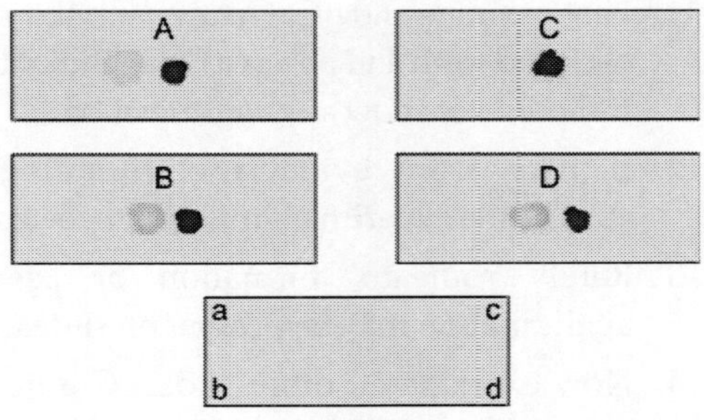

Fig. 10.1: Labelling of slides
(For color version see Plate 7)

   - Plasma factors likely to interfere with agglutination are eliminated by dilutions.
8. Now mix the antiserum with the red cell suspension on each slide by using different corners of fifth slide. Corner marked 'a' can be used for mixing antisera A with red cell suspension and similarly corners 'b' and'd' are used for mixing antisera B and antisera D. Corner marked 'c' is used for mixing red cell suspension placed as control on slide C.
9. Wait for 8-10 minutes. Then examine the slides for the presence or absence of agglutination.
10. Examination is carried both by naked eye and under microscope.
    - *Agglutination* is usually visible to naked eye. RBCs usually appear as a coarse separated red cells masses/dark red clumps of different sizes and shapes. The serum will have a brick red tinge by hemoglobin released from ruptured RBCs. On rocking the slide, clumps will not disperse.
    - *No agglutination* – The RBCs should remain separate and evenly distributed.
    - Rouleaux formation – The sedimented cells show orange tint of the red cell suspension. On rocking the slide back and forth or on blowing rouleaux formation will get dispersed while agglutinated cells will not.

11. First examine slide C. Gently rock the slide back and forth and observe for agglutination. It should not show any agglutination.
12. If there is any evidence of clumping on slide C, the experiment must be repeated.
13. Rarely rouleaux formation or pseudo agglutination may be present on slide C.
14. Now examine all other slides. Clumps of cells inseparable by shaking or blowing indicate agglutination.
15. Confirm the result under microscope. Under low power clumps are visible as dark masses and outline of RBCs cannot be seen.
16. Compare it with the control on the slide C. control is used in the experiment to avoid false-positive result.

Observation

Presence or absence of agglutination of the red cells with designated antisera indicates blood group of the individual

Agglutination on slide A	Blood group A
Agglutination on slide B	Blood group B
Agglutination on both slides A and B	Blood group AB
Agglutination on slide D	Blood group Rh+ve

ABO Blood Grouping

Slide A Antiserum A (α agglutinin)	*Slide B Antiserum B (β agglutinin)*	*Blood group*	*Agglutinogen on RBC of unknown blood sample*	*Agglutinin in plasma of unknown blood sample*
+	–	A	A	Anti-B
–	+	B	B	Anti-A
+	+	AB	AB	Nil
–	–	O		Nil

\+ Agglutination

\- No agglutination

Rh (D) Blood Grouping

Slide D Antiserum D (anti-D agglutinin)	*Blood Group*	*Agglutinogen on RBC of unknown blood sample*	*Agglutinin in plasma of unknown blood sample/ Anti-Rh antibody*
+	Rh+ve	Rh (D) antigen	Nil
–	Rh-ve	absent	Nil

\+ Agglutination

– No agglutination

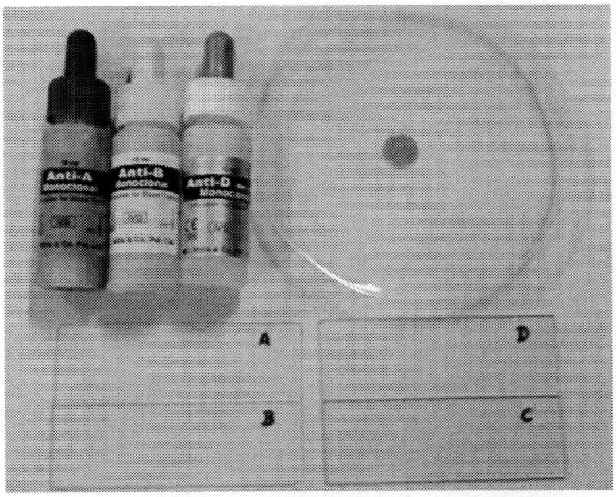

Fig. 10.2: Antiserum, watch glass and slides for blood grouping *(For color version see Plate 7)*

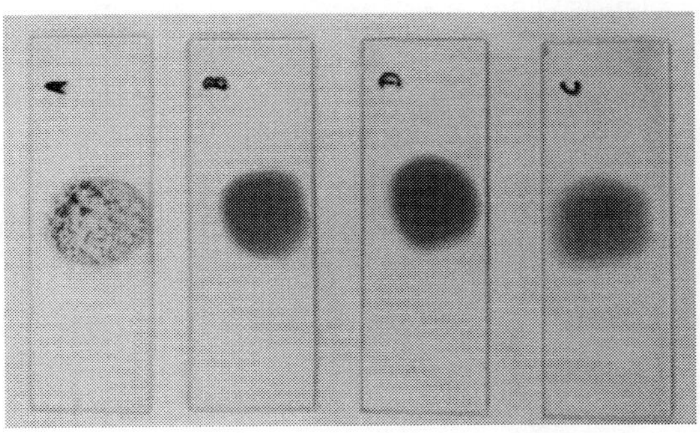

Fig. 10.3: Agglutination seen in slide A *(For color version see Plate 7)*

Sources of Error

False Positive Results are Due to

1. Rouleaux formation which should be excluded by comparing with control (red cell suspension acts as control).
2. Use of undiluted blood which may form rouleaux and give false positive results.

False Negative Results are Due to

1. Decreased immunocompetancy of antisera (because of prolonged and improper storage or expiry of sera).
2. Use of too dilute red cell suspension or addition of too small amount of red cell suspension or antisera (For agglutination reaction An-Ab (antigen-antibody) concentration has to be same, if it is not same no reaction occurs. This is called zone phenomenon.
3. Use of antisera contaminated with bacterial growth.

Precautions

1. Slide should be clean and dry to avoid hemolysis and they should be marked properly.
2. The blood should not clot before mixing with saline.
3. Never interchange the droppers of the antisera bottles.
4. Always store antisera at proper temperature when not in use.
5. Wait for 8-10 minutes before confirming presence or absence of agglutination, this time is given for An-Ab reaction to occur. If there is no clumping, wait for 15 minutes.
6. Always use diluted blood as undiluted blood may give false positive results due to rouleaux formation.
7. Do not add undiluted blood from the finger prick directly on to the antisera because the sera may get intermixed and give false positive reaction.
8. A control should always be used to exclude false +ve result.
9. Examination should be done before the preparation dries up to avoid confusion with rouleaux formation.
10. Agglutination should not be confused with clot formation.
11. Agglutination should be confirmed microscopically.
12. Clot formation, hemolysis should be excluded.

DISCUSSION

Landsteiner's Law

This law is given by Karl Landsteiner in 1900. It states that if an agglutinogen is present on the red cells of a person the corresponding agglutinin must be absent from the plasma; if agglutinogen is absent the corresponding agglutinin is present.

This law is followed by ABO system. The second part of the law is not applicable to all the blood group systems, e.g. in Rh system the absence of Rh agglutinogen (Rh negative individuals) is not accompanied by presence of anti-Rh agglutinin in the serum. Similarly, absence of M and N substance is not accompanied by presence of anti-M or anti-N agglutinins.

Clinically Important Blood Group Systems

Classical ABO system: Human beings can be divided into 4 groups according to presence or absence of different group specific substances on their surface. These group specific substances are agglutinogens (isoantigens). In the presence of suitable antibody (agglutinin) they agglutinate RBCs.

Agglutinin acting against agglutinogen A is anti-A or α agglutinin

Agglutinin acting against agglutinogen B is anti-B or β agglutinin.

Group specific substance "O" normally doesn't act as agglutinogen. There is no corresponding antibody. Very rarely after repeated transfusion group O cells evoke an irregular agglutinin, anti-O in susceptible recipients. Group O cells are not agglutinated by anti-A or anti-B antibody.

Blood group	*Group specific Substance/agglutinogen on RBCs*	*Agglutinins in plasma*
A	A	Anti-A or α
B	B	Anti-B or β
AB	A and B both	Nil
O	O	Anti-A and Anti-B

Substance A can be divided into sub groups A_1 and A_2. 75% of group A belongs to A_1 and 25% belongs to A_2.

Blood groups	*Prevalence in India (percentage)*	*Prevalence Worldwide (percentage)*
A	28	42
B	22	9
AB	5	3
O	45	46

Antigens A and B first appear at 6th week of fetal life. Concentration at birth is 1/5th of adult level then it progressively rises during puberty and adolescence. Agglutinogens A and B are not only limited to red cells but are found in many organs, e.g. Pancreas, kidney, liver, lungs, testes, salivary glands. They are water soluble and in 80% of people they appear in body secretions like saliva, semen, amniotic fluid, red cells, tears, urine. Individuals who have high concentration of these antigens in their body fluids are called **"secretors"** and those with the low concentration are called **"non secretors".**

Anti-A and anti-B agglutinins are cold antibodies they react best at 5-20°. They are IgM type. They cannot cross placenta.

Anti-D is a warm antibody. It reacts best at body temperature. It is IgG type and it can easily cross placenta.

Rh (Rhesus) System

This system was discovered by Landsteiner and Weiner in 1940. In this system there are 6 (C, D, E, c, d and e) different antigens. Among them D antigen is immunologically most significant.

Rh positive	D antigen present
Rh negative	D antigen absent

Antibody against D antigen doesn't occur naturally. The agglutinin anti-D is produced only when Rh negative individual receives Rh positive blood.

MNS and P System

The antigens of these blood groups don't evoke agglutinins in human beings. These blood groups are usually ignored for blood transfusion.

Other Blood Groups

In 1953 it was found that RBCs of 3 persons in Bombay reacted neither with anti -A, anti-B, anti-O; while their sera contained anti -A, anti-B, anti-O. This blood group has called as Bombay group. Some of the other blood groups are Lewis, Lutheran, Kell, Duffy, Kidd, etc.

Blood Group Determination is Indicated for:

1. Blood transfusion.
2. Determination of Rh incompatibility between mother and child.
3. For settling paternity disputes. By blood grouping (ABO, Rh, MNS) it is possible to prove that a person could not be the father, but not that he is the father.
4. Choice of a donor in tissue or organ transplant.
5. Genetic studies.
6. Medico legal cases.
7. Determining the susceptibility to disease e.g. blood group O people are more susceptible to peptic ulcer and blood group A people are more susceptible to carcinoma of stomach and diabetes mellitus.

Blood Transfusion

Blood transfusion is required in the cases of

1. Accidents.
2. Surgery.
3. Preoperatively to build up patient.
4. Patients having blood disorders like severe anemia, leukemia, hemophilia, purpura.
5. Shock.
6. CO poisoning.

Prerequisites of Blood Transfusion

1. Blood grouping – ABO and Rh grouping.
2. Cross matching – Minor and major.
3. Screening of blood for the presence of any blood transmitted diseases.
4. Selecting a good donor – One who is between 18-60 years of age with normal Hb levels. Pregnant and lactating mothers should be excluded. Professional donors should be discouraged.

Minor Cross Matching

The donor's plasma is matched against red cells of the recipient. It is slightly less important as compared to major cross matching because antibodies present in small amount of donor's plasma will get diluted with the recipient's plasma. Secondly they will also get neutralized by the soluble agglutinogens present in the recipient's plasma. Minor cross matching cannot be totally ignored because if the agglutinin titre of the donor's cells is more it may agglutinate recipient's cells.

Major Cross Matching

The cells of donor (agglutinogens) are directly matched against the plasma agglutinins of recipient. It is important to ensure that the antibodies present in the recipient's plasma don't agglutinate donor's cells.

Universal Donor and Universal Recipient

O-negative blood persons are considered as universal donors and 'AB+ve' persons are considered as universal recipient.

Autologous Transfusion

Transfusion of once own blood is called autologous transfusion. It is usually practised for elective surgeries. Persons blood is collected few days prior to surgery and stored for future use (transfused during or after the surgery). This procedure avoids the risks of transmission of AIDS, hepatitis, etc.

WORK SPACE

Name of subject
Age

Sex

Reaction of subject's blood with

Antiserum – A	*Antiserum – B*	*Antiserum – D*	*Blood group*

Agglutination "+"
No agglutination "–"

ANSWER THESE QUESTIONS

Q1. Enumerate the hazards of missmatched blood transfusion.

Q2. What happens if a Rh-ve mother carries a Rh+ve fetus?

VIVA QUESTIONS

Q 1. What is the importance of using control?

Q2. How will you differentiate agglutination from rouleaux formation?

Q3. Why we should wait for 8-10 minutes before looking for agglutination?

Q4. Why ABO incompatibility between a mother and a foetus rarely cause any problem?

Q5. What are the indications of blood grouping?

Q6. What are the indications of blood transfusion?

CHAPTER

11

Determination of Bleeding Time (BT) and Clotting Time (CT)

OBJECTIVES

After completing the practical student should:

- Be able to define BT and CT.
- Know the clinical importance of BT and CT.
- Know different methods for determining BT and CT.
- Determine BT by Duke's method and CT by capillary glass tube method.
- Know the precautions observed in each method.
- Be able to describe the physiological basis of bleeding disorders.
- Be able to name the conditions in which BT or CT is increased.

INTRODUCTION

Any kind of trauma to blood vessel leads to bleeding which stops spontaneously by a process called hemostasis. Frequent and pro-longed bleeding with small injuries or even spontaneous bleeding without any injury warrants investigation. In such cases bleeding and clotting times are determined to assess the integrity of hemostatic mechanisms.

DETERMINATION OF BT

Bleeding time: It is the time from the onset of bleeding till the (unassisted) stoppage of bleeding.

Tests for Determination of Bleeding Time (BT)

1. Duke's method
2. Ivy's method
3. Simplate method

DUKE'S METHOD

It is the most frequently used method in clinical labs as it is very easy to perform and minimal equipment and laboratory skill is required.

Principle

A deep skin puncture is made and the length of time required for bleeding to stop is recorded.

Apparatus

1. Equipment for sterile skin prick.
2. Whatman filter paper.
3. Stopwatch.

Procedure

1. Thoroughly clean the finger tip or ear lobe with spirit swab and allow it to dry.
2. With a sterile lancet make a 3-4 mm deep skin puncture on the finger tip to get free flowing blood.
3. Immediately start the stopwatch.
4. After 30 seconds blot the drop of blood coming out of the incision on the filter paper edge.

5. Blot subsequent drops after every 30 seconds a little further along the filter paper.
6. When no further blood spot appears on the filter paper, i.e. when bleeding ceases, stop the stopwatch.
7. Count, encircle and number the blood spots on the filter paper.
8. Keep this piece of filter paper and paste it in your work space.

Observations

Note that after every 30 seconds the drop formed will be smaller than the previous one.

Calculation and result:

Multiply the total number of blood spots by 30 seconds. It will give you the reading of the bleeding time by this method.

Normal bleeding time by Duke's method is 1-5 minutes (1-3 min for finger tip prick, 3-5 min for ear lobe prick).

Precautions

1. Do not rub too much while cleaning finger tip as rubbing increases blood flow and alters BT.

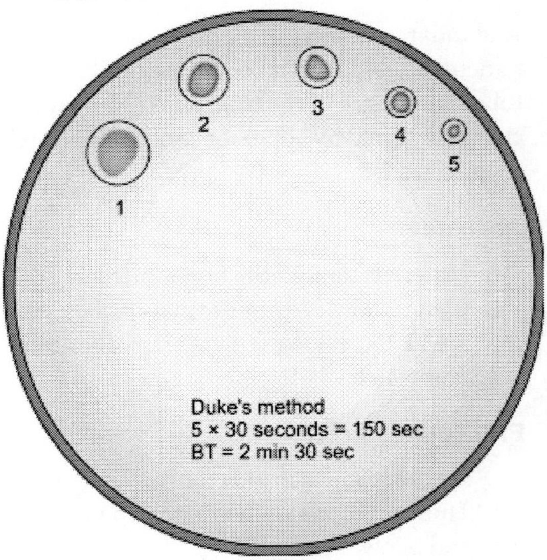

Fig. 11.1: Duke method of determining BT

2. Skin should be completely dry before pricking.
3. Finger should be pricked by a single stabbing action to give free flowing blood.
4. Skin puncture should be 3-4 mm deep.
5. Finger tip should not be squeezed after it has been pricked.
6. Immediately start the stop watch as soon as the finger is pricked.
7. Do not press the pricked finger on the filter paper as it may interfere in bleeding instead blot the blood drop lightly.
8. If bleeding does not stop in 10 minutes discontinue the test and apply pressure over the wound to stop bleeding.

IVY'S METHOD

This method is more reliable and standardized than the Duke's method but it is more painful to the subject and more skill is required to perform it.

Principle

Standard incisions are made on the forearm and the length of time required for bleeding to cease is recorded.

Apparatus

1. Equipment for sterile skin puncture.
2. Filter papers.
3. Sphygmomanometer.
4. Stopwatch.

Procedure

1. Tie the Sphygmomanometer cuff on the upper arm of the subject.
2. Clean anterior surface of forearm with spirit.
3. Apply pressure of 40 mm Hg and maintain this pressure till the end of the experiment.
4. Hold the skin tightly by grasping the underside of forearm.

5. With the sterilized needle make two (3 mm) deep skin punctures 5 mm apart on the anterior aspect of the forearm of the subject about 5-6 cm below the cubital fossa.
6. Immediately start the stop watch.
7. After every 30 seconds, blot the blood oozing out of two punctured sites on the edges of two separate filter papers.
8. When the bleeding stops stop the stopwatch.
9. Record the bleeding time of both the punctures. The longer of the two bleeding times will be the final reading.

   Normal bleeding time by this method is 3-8 minutes.

Precautions

1. Puncture site should be properly cleaned.
2. Two punctures should be given in quick succession.
3. A constant pressure of 40 mm Hg should be maintained through out the procedure.
4. Though it is difficult to control the depth of the puncture but it should be around 3 mm deep.
5. Take care not to puncture any superficial vein.
6. The longer of the bleeding times should be taken for the result.

SIMPLATE METHOD

The difficulty to control the depth of the puncture faced in Duke's and Ivy's method is over come with this technique. A template or automated scalpel is used to control the length (9 mm) and depth (1 mm) of the wound.

Apparatus

1. Equipment for sterile skin prick.
2. Automated scalpel.
3. Filter paper.
4. Sphygmomanometer.
5. Stopwatch.

Procedure and Precautions

Similar to Ivy's method. Normal bleeding time by this method is < 7 minutes.

DETERMINATION OF CT

Clotting time: It is the time from the onset of bleeding till the clot formation.

Tests for Determination of Clotting Time (CT)

1. Wright's capillary glass tube method
2. Lee and white method

WRIGHT'S CAPILLARY GLASS TUBE METHOD

It is the most convenient and commonly used method in practice. It requires minimal skill. It tests both the intrinsic (contact of the blood with glass capillary) and extrinsic (tissue trauma leading to admixture of blood with tissue fluid which contains thromboplastin) mechanism of clotting.

Principle

A standard incision is made in the skin of the patient and blood is taken into a capillary glass tube. The length of the time it takes for blood to clot (as detected by appearance of fibrin string) is reported as CT.

Apparatus

1. Materials for a sterile finger prick.
2. Clean and dry thin capillary tubes which are 12-15 cm long with 1-2 mm diameter.
3. Stopwatch.

Procedure

1. Set the stopwatch at zero.
2. Thoroughly clean the finger tip with spirit and allow it to dry.

3. Make a 3 mm deep prick with a sterile lancet to get free flowing blood.
4. Immediately start the stopwatch.
5. Discard the first drop of blood and allow a large drop of blood to form.
6. Fill the capillary tube by dipping its one end into the drop and lowering the other end. Blood will flow rapidly into the tube by capillary action.
7. Hold the filled capillary tube between the palms of your hands so as to maintain it at body temperature.
8. After 1 minute, gently break off capillary tube 1 cm bit from one end. Thereafter break 1 cm bit of capillary tube after every 30 seconds and look for appearance of fibrin thread.
9. When a thin string (5 mm in length) of fibrin is seen between the broken ends, stop the watch and note the time.

Observation

After sometime of filling the capillary a thin string of fibrin 5 mm in length is seen between its broken ends.

The total time taken from the time of puncture till the formation of fibrin thread is the CT.

Normal value of CT by this method is 2-8 minutes.

Precautions

1. Take all the precautions for pricking.
2. Skin puncture should be 3 mm deep and blood should flow spontaneously.
3. Discard the first drop.
4. Pricked finger should not be squeezed.
5. Stopwatch should be started immediately as soon as the blood first appears.
6. Glass capillary tube should never be filled with blood by means of sucking at its other end.
7. Immediately after filling, the capillary tube should be held between the palms to maintain it at body temperature. Temperature affects clotting.
8. After every 30 seconds look for the formation of fibrin thread.

LEE AND WHITE TEST TUBE METHOD

This is more reliable and sensitive than the capillary method but needs more special arrangements. It tests the intrinsic system of blood clotting.

Principle

Venous blood is collected in a clean glass test tube. The time taken for blood to clot at 37°C is noted as CT.

Apparatus

1. Disposable needle with a syringe.
2. Methylated spirit.
3. Three test tubes.
4. Waterbath.
5. Stopwatch.

Procedure

1. Under aseptic conditions collect 5 ml of venous blood by nontraumatic venipuncture.
2. Start the stopwatch as soon as the blood starts entering the syringe.
3. Remove the needle from the syringe and add 1.5 ml blood in each of the three test tubes.
4. Place these test tubes in a waterbath at 37°C
5. After one minute, take out the first test tube from the waterbath and tilt it at an angle of 45° to check whether blood has clotted and there is no spillage of blood on tilting.
6. If the blood doesn't spill on tilting note the time but if it spills, return it to water bath.
7. Repeat it after every 30 seconds until the test tube can be tilted without spilling blood.

8. Once the blood in first test tube clots note the time and take out second test tube.
9. Repeat the tilting on the second test tube to see for the spillage of blood (which usually occurs a little after the first test tube because tilting has hastened the CT in first test tube). If there is no spillage, stop the stopwatch and note the time.
10. The CT is the clotting time in second test tube.
11. The third test tube acts as a control and a check on the end point in the second tube.

    Normal value of CT by this method is 5-12 minutes.

Precautions

1. Take all aseptic precautions.
2. Venipuncture should be non traumatic.
3. Air bubbles should not enter the syringe. They shorten the CT.
4. Don't take less than 1 ml of blood in test tubes otherwise it will give false low reading.
5. CT of second test tube should be taken as the final reading.
6. Temperature of tubes should be maintained at 37°C throughout the test.

DISCUSSION

Indications of Determining BT and CT

BT and CT are important in the following situations:

1. If a person has history of frequent and persistent bleeding from minor injuries/ spontaneous bleeding into tissues.
2. Before any minor/major surgery (this includes tooth extraction also).
3. Before taking biopsy especially from bone marrow, liver, kidney, etc.
4. Before and during anticoagulant therapy.
5. If there is family history of bleeding disorders.

Bleeding Disorders

Excessive bleeding with small injuries or spontaneous bleeding may result from abnormalities of:

i. Platelets
ii. Blood vessel walls
iii. Coagulation defects

Platelets and Vessel Wall Defects

Typically cause bleeding from small vessels during cuts and bruises and bleeding in gums.

Coagulation Defects

Defects of coagulation includes:

i. Conditions characterized by excessive bleeding into tissues, muscles, joints which usually occur due to trauma to a large vessel. The delay in formation of a clot fails to check blood loss.
ii. Clotting of blood within unbroken blood vessels which is known as thrombosis.

BT and CT are done together in all disorders of hemostasis. Platelets are involved in both tests.

BT tests the Platelets Plug Formation and the Condition of the Micro Vessels.

BT Depends on

1. Status of the vessel wall and platelet count.
2. Temperature: In cold weather, low temperature promotes vasoconstriction.

BT Gets Prolonged in

1. *Thrombocytopenia:* Low platelet count (less than 50,000/µl of blood) may be caused by:
   - Decreased production of platelets due to bone marrow depression caused by
     - irradiation, cytotoxic drugs, sulpha drugs or chloramphenicol
     - septicemia and aplastic anemia

  - leukemias, malignant invasion of bone marrow.
- Increased destruction of platelets caused by
  - Disseminated intravascular coagulation: It is a hemorrhagic disorder in which diffuse intravascular clotting causes hemostatic defect resulting from utilization of clotting factors and platelets in the clotting process. It may be caused by mismatched transfusion reaction, gram-negative or meningococcal septicemia, hypersensitivity reactions, obstetrical accidents (like abruptio placenta, amniotic fluid embolism, retention of dead fetus), etc.
  - Certain drugs: Quinine, quinidine, thiazides, methyl dopa, and estrogens.
  - Autoimmune destruction of platelets: As seen in idiopathic thrombocytopenic purpura.
  - destruction of platelets due to hypersplenism.
  - Increased sequestration of platelets in enlarged spleen.

2. *Thromboasthenia:* Platelet count is normal but platelets are functionally abnormal, e.g. thrombasthenic purpura.
3. *Von Willebrand disease:* Platelet defect combined with a component of factor VIII deficiency.
4. *Vessel wall defects:* This includes inherited-idiopathic purpura and acquired purpura. Acquired purpura can occur due to —
   - drugs like corticosteroids, aspirin, penicillins and sulpha drugs,
   - allergic reactions
   - old age (senile purpura)
   - Connective tissue diseases
   - Infections like subacute bacterial endocarditis, typhus or meningococcal infection
   - Deficiency of vitamin C
   - Diseases like uremia, cirrhosis, leukemias, etc.

VON WILLEBRAND DISEASE

It is an inherited autosomal dominant (occasionally recessive) hemostatic disorder. It affects both the sexes. Usually there is mild degree of bleeding tendency leading to easy bruisability; mucosal bleeding, epistaxisis, increased bleeding after mild trauma. This disease is characterized by prolonged BT due to deficiency of a component of factor VIII (which along with ADP is responsible for platelet adhesion).

PURPURA

This disease is characterized by prolonged BT. The patient will have petechial hemorrhages and easy bruisability. According to the cause it can be primary or secondary.

- Primary purpura: It is idiopathic and inherited. There is anatomical defect in vessel walls, they fail to contract normally
- Secondary purpura: There is no structural deformity of vessel walls. It is secondary to some cause like drugs, antigen-antibody reaction, allergic reactions, old age (senile purpura)
- Thrombocytopenic purpura: Purpura due to platelet
- Purpura due to decrease platelet function – thrombasthenic purpura
- Purpura due to antibodies formed against platelets – immune thrombocytopenic purpura

CT Tests the Formation of the Clot

If CT is > 15 min, patient should be subjected to detailed investigations to identify missing coagulation factors.

CT Depends on

1. Temperature – Low temperature may prolong CT
2. Presence and absence of clotting factors

CT Gets Prolonged in

1. Hemophilia
2. Christmas disease
3. Afibrogenemia/dysfibrogenemia
4. Deficiency of any clotting factor
5. Liver diseases
6. Vitamin K deficiency
7. DIC
8. Overdose of anticoagulant therapy

HEMOPHILIA

It is a disease where CT is prolonged but BT remains normal. There is tendency to bleed from nose, mucosal surfaces, subcutaneous tissues, muscles, joints. Bleeding occurs spontaneously or after mild trauma. It is an X-linked inherited disorder (males are sufferers, females are carriers). *Hemophilia-A* is also called classical hemophilia. It is caused by the deficiency of factor VIII. *Hemophilia-B* is also called Christmas disease is due to deficiency of factor IX.

WORK SPACE

Name Age

Sex Date

BT by Duke's method=

CT by capillary glass tube method=

ANSWER THESE QUESTIONS

Q1. Define BT and give its various methods of determination.

Q2. What is the normal value of BT by Duke's method?

Q3. What are the indications for doing BT and CT?

Q4. Name the conditions where BT is prolonged?

Q5. **Define CT and give its various methods of determination.**

Q6. **What is the normal value of CT by capillary glass tube method?**

Q7. **Name the conditions where CT is prolonged.**

VIVA QUESTIONS

Q1. Which is the most reliable method for determining BT and why?

Q2. What precautions are taken for determining BT by Duke's method?

Q3. What are the factors on which BT depends?

Q4. What is Purpura?

Q5. What is Hemophilia?

Q6. Which is the most reliable method for determining CT?

Q7. What precautions are to be taken for determining CT by capillary glass tube method?

Q8. What are the factors affecting CT?

Q9. Enumerate clotting factors.

Demonstration Section 2

CHAPTER

12

Determination of Packed Cell Volume/Hematocrit

DEMONSTRATION-1

OBJECTIVE

After completing demonstration student should:

- Be able to define hematocrit
- Know different methods of PCV determination
- Know three layers obtained on centrifuging blood by wintrobes method
- Know normal levels of hematocrit
- Know the uses of PCV determination
- Know different blood indices.

INTRODUCTION

Hematocrit (Hct) is the volume of red blood cells expressed as a percentage of volume of whole blood in a blood sample. Hct is also called packed cell volume. The plasma is separated from the formed elements of the blood and the percentage of volume of the packed red cells is measured.

METHODS OF DETERMINATION

1. Manual method
   - Macrohematocrit method/Wintrobe method
   - Microhemarocrit method
2. Automated method

AUTOMATED METHOD

It is done by using electronic cell counters.

Result obtained is more accurate, as the result is computed from individual red cell volumes so it is not affected by trapped plasma left in red cell column.

MANUAL METHOD (WINTROBE METHOD)

Principle

A sample of blood to which an anticoagulant has been added is taken in a hematocrit tube and centrifuged. RBCs (sp gravity = 1.090) and other cellular elements of blood being heavier than plasma (sp gravity = 1.030) gets packed towards the bottom of tube by the centrifugal force and the plasma is separated. The volume occupied by the red blood cells is measured and its ratio with the volume of whole blood is calculated.

Apparatus

1. Disposable syringe with needle.
2. Spirit Swab.
3. Anticoagulant: Double oxalate or EDTA
4. Pasteur pipette: It is a 22 cm long glass pipette with a thin 14 cm long nozzle. A rubber teat is provided to suck blood into

the pipette. It is used to transfer blood from the container to Wintrobe's tube.

5. Wintrobe's tube: It's a thick walled 11 cm long tube with uniform bore of 2 mm. It is calibrated in cms and mms. From above downwards the markings from 0 to 10 cm on one side of the scale are for ESR and 10 to 0 cm on other side of the scale for Hct. It can hold 1 ml of blood sample.
6. Centrifuge machine: It is used to induce centrifugal force to pack blood cells in the wintrobe tube. The magnitude of centrifugal force created depends upon–
   - The radius, i.e. the distance between the center of the shaft and the bottom of the centrifuge tube when it has been laid horizontally
   - The number of revolutions/min.

The centrifuge should be capable of producing a force of 2300 g. In terms of G, i.e. gravitational force, the value of centrifugal force created should be 2300 units. This much force is created if the radius is 22.5 cm and speed is 3000 revolutions/min.

Force of < 2300g – will give false high Hct reading

Force of > 2300g – will give false low Hct values

Procedure

1. Under aseptic condition draw around 2 ml of venous blood.
2. Transfer it to a vial containing anticoagulant (double oxalate). Mix it well by repeated inversions or rotating the vial between hands.
3. Fill the Pasteur pipette carefully with blood. Insert the tip of pipette to the bottom of Wintrobe's tube and fill it from bottom by gradually withdrawing the pipette upwards keeping the tip under the rising column of blood.
4. Fill the Wintrobe's tube till 10 cm mark. If more blood is accidentally added remove it with the help of dropper.
5. If less blood is added, add more and bring the volume to 10 cm mark. If no more blood is available. Fill the tube with all that is available.
6. Place the Wintrobe's tube containing sample in one of the cups of the centrifuge

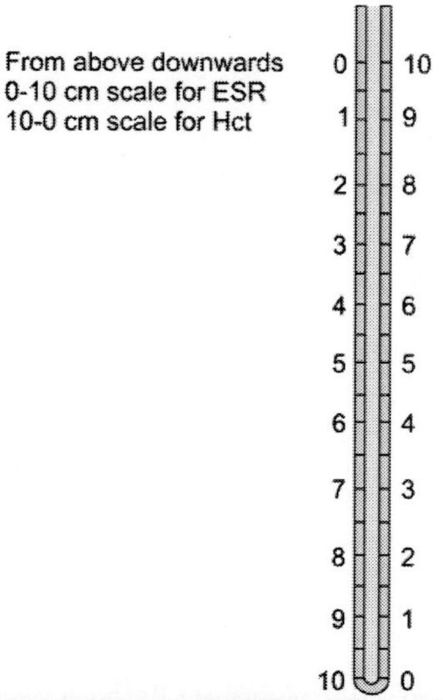

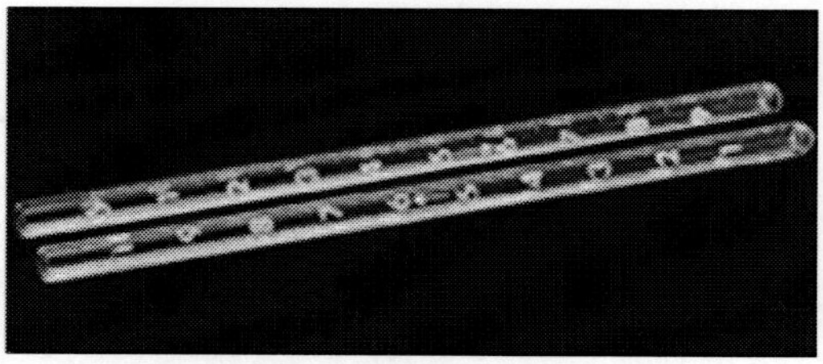

Fig. D1.1: Wintrobe's tubes

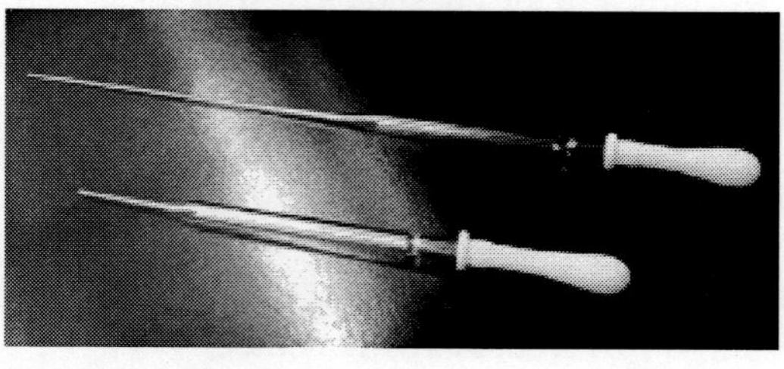

Fig. D1.2: Pasteur pipette *(For color version see Plate 7)*

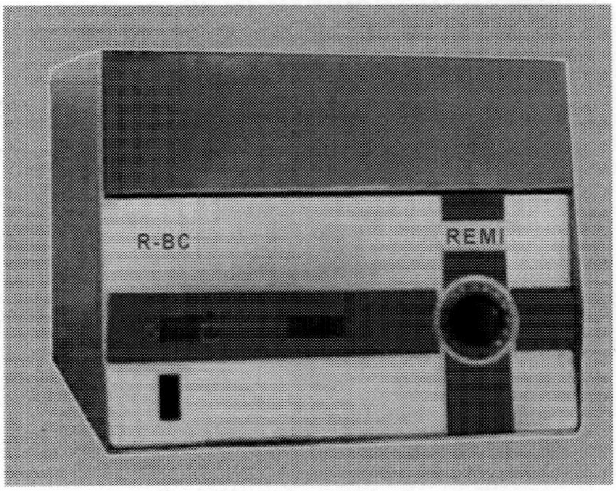

Fig. D1.3: Centrifuge

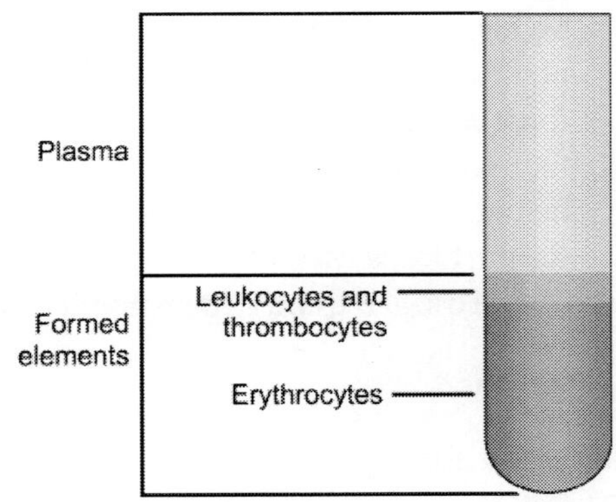

Fig. D1.4: Separation of blood sample in three layers

and another Wintrobe's tube containing water in opposite cup of centrifuge to balance it.

7. Centrifuge the sample first at slow speed then gradually increase the speed to 3000 rpm for 30 minutes.
8. After 30 minutes switch off the centrifuge and allow it to stop by itself. Do not use the brake.
9. Take out the tube and record observation.

Observations

The blood sample will be separated into 3 layers.

1. The top layer of clear straw colored plasma.
2. Middle layer is thin 0.5-1 mm grayish white layer called "buffy coat/layer." It consists of platelets above and leukocytes below.
3. A bottom layer of red cells with its upper level distinctly visible and sharp. There is a grayish line separating WBCs from the red cell layer. This line is due to presence of reduced Hb in the RBCs lying adjacent to the WBCs which reduce the oxyHb. The line marks the upper limit of RBC layer. The height of RBC layer is normally between 4.2-4.7 cm.
4. The percentage of the height of the column of blood occupied by packed red cells constitutes the Hct or the packed cell volume.

Calculation

1. If the blood sample taken is upto 10 mark PCV percentage is given by multiplying the reading obtained by 10, e.g. If the reading obtained is 4.2

$$\text{Hct} = 4.2 \times 10 = 42\%$$

2. If the sample is not upto 10 cm mark, then Hct is—

$$\frac{\text{Height of packed red cells in mm}}{\text{Height of packed cells \& plasma in mm (height of whole sample)}} \quad 100$$

Result

1. Take the reading of packed red cells, centrifuge the tube again for 5 minute and note the readings.
2. Repeat if there is difference in Hct value.
3. Take final reading when 3 consecutive readings (at 5 min intervals) are identical.

Precautions

1. PCV should be determined within 6 hours of sample collection (or the sample should

be kept in refrigerator) otherwise the change in red cell metabolism will cause changes in RBC size and shape. Hemolysis will also start after 6 hours. This will give wrong Hct reading.

2. Mix blood thoroughly with correct amount of anticoagulant before taking sample for PCV determination. Excess anticoagulant if used will cause hemolysis and give false low Hct.
3. Do not use hemolysed specimen it will give false low reading.
4. The vial containing anticoagulant and blood should be rotated between palms to ensure oxygenation of RBCs and to remove CO_2. If it is not done it can give false high reading because in venous blood high CO_2 increases red cell size.
5. While filling the Wintrobe's tube to avoid air bubble formation and damage to red cells, the pasteur pipette should be withdrawn gradually keeping its tip under the rising column of blood.
6. There should be no air bubble in the tube and if it is present discard that sample.
7. Wintrobe's tube should not be filled from the top as blood will not flow down to its bottom (because of air present in the tube).
8. Excess amount of blood if present in the tube shall be removed by dropper, not with any absorbent material.

Advantages of Wintrobe's Method

1. ESR and PCV can both be determined by using the same sample.
2. It is inexpensive method.

Sources of Error

1. Inadequate mixing of blood.
2. Improper concentration of anticoagulant.
3. Irregular bore of tube.
4. Inadequate centrifugation leading to incomplete packing of cells.

MICROHEMATOCRIT METHOD

Principle

Anticoagulated blood is centrifuged in a sealed capillary tube, volume of packed red cells and percentage of whole blood are determined by a special hematocrit reader.

Apparatus

1. Disposable lancet.
2. Spirit swab.
3. Heparinized capillary hematocrit tubes: These are about 75 mm long with internal diameter of 1 mm.
4. Microhematocrit Centrifuge: It is a special high speed centrifuge that runs at a speed of 12000 rpm. It is capable of producing force of 12000 g.
5. Hematocrit reader: Several types of hematocrit readers are available they have scale which is used for reading PCV.
6. Clay: To seal the end of hematocrit tubes.

Procedure

1. Under aseptic conditions prick the finger tip.
2. Fill three quarters of two heparinized capillary tube with the blood.
3. Seal the dry end of the tube with plastic sealing clay.
4. Place them in radial grooves of centrifuge, with their heads opposite each other.
5. Centrifuge for 5 minute at 12000 rpm.
6. Take out tubes and read the PCV from microhematocrit reader.

Precautions

Same as for macrohematocrit method

Advantages

1. Very little blood is need. So it can be used in pediatric patients.

2. It is less time consuming.
3. It can be used for mass surveys because large number of samples can be handled simultaneously.

Normal Values

Males	–	47·7%
Females	–	42·5%
Full term baby/newborn	–	54·10%
Infants	–	38·6%
Children	–	41·4%

DISCUSSION

True Hematocrit

With manual method about 2% plasma remains entrapped between the cells. The percentage is more if RBCs are abnormal in shape, e.g. spherocytes in sickle cell anemia. True hematocrit is Hct without entrapped plasma. To get true hematocrit (i.e. without entrapped plasma), multiply observed Hct with 0.98.

Whole Body Hct

Hct of venous blood is higher than that of microcirculation (due to axial streaming of RBCs) and arterial blood (RBCs are larger in venous blood). To calculate whole body Hct from observed value multiply that with 0.87.

Uses of Hct Determination

1. It is used for detecting the presence and degree of anemia and polycythemia.
2. Hct is a more reliable of the Red cell population in the blood than manually estimated RBC count, because much less error is associated with Hct determination.
3. If Hct is determined by Wintrobe's method one can obtain additional information, e.g.
   - Buffy coat thickness of 1 mm implies TLC of about 10000
   - Absent or minimal buffy coat implies leucopenia
   - Buffy coat >1 mm implies leukocytosis
   - In subleukemic leukemia film can be made from buffy cell layer where high concentration of WBCs are available. Identification of typical cells will become easier and less time consuming.
   - For LE cell phenomenon test WBCs can also be picked up from buffy coat.
   - The changed color of plasma layer can give important information, e.g.
     - Yellow colored plasma ...... jaundice
     - Pink colored plasma .... hemolysis
     - Creamy white plasma ...... increased chylomicrons/hyperlipidemia
     - Brownish plasma methalbuminemia.
4. If Hb Concentration, RBC count and PCV are known, various absolute blood values and indices of a person can be calculated. These indices are important for morphological classifications of anemias. There are different blood indices like MCV, MCH, and MCHC.

Blood Indices which are Important for Morphological Classification of Anemias

MCV: Mean corpuscular volume.

It is the average volume of a single RBC. It is expressed in femtoliters.

$$\text{MCV} = \frac{\text{PCV}}{\text{RBC count in millions / mm}^3} \quad 10$$

$$= \frac{45 \quad 10}{5} \quad 90\ \text{fl}$$

Normal MCV value – 78-96 fl (femtoliters)

If MCV is more than normal cell RBC are macrocytes as seen in megaloblastic anemias.

MCV value	RBC called as
Normal	Normocytes
High	Macrocytes
low	Microcytes

MCH: Mean corpuscular Hb

It is the average amount of Hb in a single RBC. It is expressed in picograms.

$$\text{MCH} = \frac{\text{Hb in gm\%}}{\text{RBC count in millions / mm}^3} \quad 10$$

$$= \frac{15\%}{5 \text{ millions / mm}^3} \quad 10 \quad 30 \text{ pg}$$

Normal MCH value – 27-33 pg (picograms)

MCHC: Mean corpuscular Hb concentration.

It represents the relationship between the cell volume and its degree of saturation with Hb. MCHC doesn't consider RBC count but represents the actual Hb concentration of red cells only. It is expressed in percentage

$$\text{MCHC} = \frac{\text{Hb in gm\%}}{\text{PCV}} \quad 100$$

$$= \frac{15}{45} \quad 100 \quad 33.33\%$$

Normal MCHC value – 30-37%

MCHC levels can never exceed 37% because this is the upper limit of Hb concentrating ability of RBCs. The Hb synthesizing machinery of RBCs doesn't have the Hb concentrating capacity beyond this limit.

MCHC value	RBC
Normal	Normochromic
Low	Hypochromic

Anemia Classification Based on Blood Indices

RBC	Normochromic	Hypochromic
Normocytic	Acute hemorrhagic anemia Hemolytic anemias (except thalassemia) Aplastic anemia	Chronic hemorrhagic anemia
Macrocytic	B12 and folic acid deficiency anemia	Anemia secondary to liver disease
Microcytic	Anemia after chronic infections	Iron deficiency anemia Thalassemia

Conditions which alter PCV/Hct

Increase in Hct

Physiological

1. Due to increased RBC count:
   - High altitude
   - Newborns
   - Males as compared to females.
2. Due to change in plasma volume or redistribution of cells:
   - Excessive sweating
   - Severe exercise
   - Emotional stress.

Pathological

1. Due to increased RBC count:
   - Polycythemia rubra Vera
   - Hypoxia due to congenital heart disease or lung disease.
2. Due to change in plasma volume:
   - Vomiting
   - Diarrhea.

Decrease in Hct

Physiological

1. Pregnancy
2. Females as compared to males
3. Excessive water intake.

Pathological

1. Anemias
2. Bone marrow depression
3. Hyperaldosteronism.

WORK SPACE

ANSWER THESE QUESTIONS

Q1. What is hematocrit or packed cell volume?

Q2. What is true Hematocrit?

Q3. What is buffy layer? Give its importance.

Q4. What is the significance of determining PCV?

VIVA QUESTIONS

Q1. What are the different methods of determining PCV?

Q2. Why it is important to determine PCV within 6 hrs of sample collection?

Q3. What is the normal value of PCV in adults?

Q4. Give various conditions which alter PCV.

Q5. Why PCV is higher in venous blood?

CHAPTER

13

Determination of Erythrocyte Sedimentation Rate (ESR)

DEMONSTRATION-2

OBJECTIVE

After completing demonstration student should:

- Be able to define ESR
- Know about various methods of measuring ESR
- Know the precautions observed
- Know about the Clinical uses of ESR determination.

INTRODUCTION

ESR is a simple non-specific screening test that indirectly measures the presence of inflammation in the body. It reflects the tendency of red blood cells to settle more rapidly in the face of some disease states, usually because of increases in plasma fibrinogen, immuno-globulins, and other acute-phase reaction proteins.

Principle

When anticoagulated whole blood is allowed to stand in a narrow vertical tube for a period of time, the RBCs under the influence of gravity settle down from the plasma. The rate at which they settle is measured as the number of millimetres of RBC column present below the column of clear plasma after one hour (mm/hr).

Methods

Many test methods are commercially available for performing the ESR. Each method has its own characteristics, and the results from different ESR methods should not be considered interchangeable. Most testing are done with—

1. Westergren method
2. Wintrobe Method.

WESTERGREN METHOD

Most laboratories use the Westergren method

Apparatus

1. Mathylated spiriti cotton, sterile gauze.
2. 2 ml syringe.
3. Vial.
4. 3.8% Sodium citrate: Used as anticoagulant, 1 part of anticoagulant is added to 4 parts of blood.
5. Westergren pipette: It is 30 cm long pipette (open at both the ends) with the bore diameter of 2.5 mm. The lower 20 cms are calibrated from 0-200 mm from top to bottom. It holds 1 ml of blood.
6. Westergren stand: It can hold around 6 Westergren pipettes at a time. To hold

Westergren pipettes in the vertical position it has rubber pad at the lower end and screws at the upper end.

Procedure

1. Under aseptic precautions collect 2 ml of venous blood.
2. Transfer it into a vail containing 0 .5 ml of sodium citrate.
3. Mix the blood with anticoagulant by inverting the vial.
4. Draw blood into Westergren pipette up to the 0 mm mark. Immediately close the upper end of the pipette with the thumb to prevent blood from running down.
5. Place the lower end of the pipette on the rubber pad of the rack, fix it vertically in the rack with the help of screws provided on the upper end of the rack.
6. Let it stand in strictly vertical position for 1 hour at room temperature.
7. After one hour note the reading, i.e. the level to which red cell column has fallen.

Observation

1. After one hour red cells being heavier (sp gravity 1.095) than plasma (sp gravity 1.032) would have settled down below the column of plasma.
2. Note the reading corresponding to the upper limit of the red cell sediment. This will give the value of ESR.

Result

The distance of fall of erythrocytes, expressed as millimeters in 1st hour.

ESR is expressed as .... mm/hr

Precautions

1. Sample should be collected in fasting state.
2. Proper amount of anticoagulant should be used and mixed properly with blood. If higher concentration of anticoagulant is added it will give false low value.
3. Sample should be stored no longer than 2 hours at room temperature or 6 hours at 4°C.
4. There should be no air bubble in the pipette and it should be filled up to zero mark.
5. Pipette should be kept vertical and undisturbed for 1 hour. Any tilting will give false high reading.
6. Test should be done at room temperature. High temperature gives false high value and low temperature gives false low reading of ESR.
7. Reading should be taken after 1 hour (not after ½ hr and multiplying by 2) because the rate of sedimentation is slow in the beginning and becomes fast only after 45 minutes. 95-98% RBCs settle down by the end of 1 hour.

Advantages of Westergren Method

It has an advantage that highly elevated ESR can be detected due to the tall column height of the Westergren pipette.

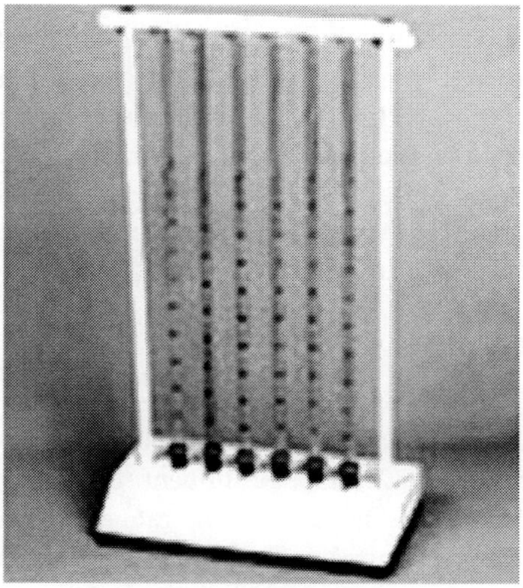

Fig. D2.1: Westergren stand with pipettes

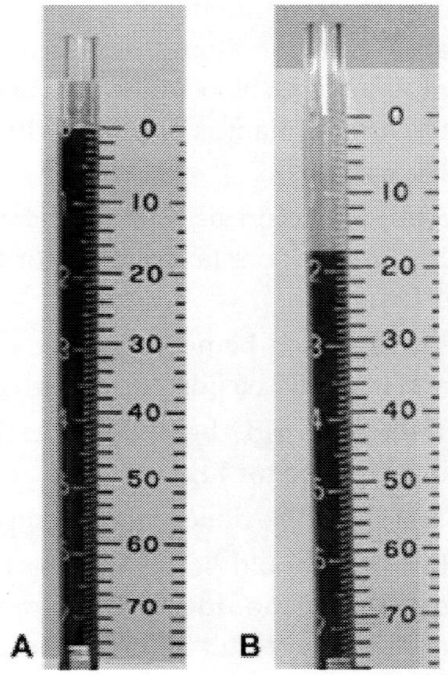

Fig. D2.2: Westergren pipettes, A – at the start of test and B – after 1 hour showing clear plasma column above and RBC column below. ESR reading 22 mm in first hour

Normal Value by This Method

Males: 3-5 mm at the end of 1st hour
Females: 5-12 at the end of 1st hour

WINTROBE METHOD

Apparatus

1. Material for collecting venous blood under aseptic conditions.
2. 2 ml syringe.
3. Vial.
4. Double oxalate or EDTA as anticoagulant.
   - Pasteur pipette: It is a 22 cm long glass pipette with a thin 14 cm long nozzle. A rubber teat is provided to suck blood into the pipette. It is used to transfer blood from the vial to fill Wintrobe tube.
5. Wintrobe tube: It is a thick walled 11 cm long tube with uniform bore of 2 mm. It is calibrated in cms and mms. From above downwards the markings from 0 to 10 cm on one side of the scale are for ESR.
6. Wintrobe stand: It is a stand for holding Wintrobe tubes in vertical position.

Procedure

1. Under aseptic condition draw around 2 ml of venous blood.
2. Transfer it to a vial containing anti-coagulant (double oxalate). Mix it well by repeated inversions or rotating the vial between hands.
3. Fill the pasteur pipette carefully with blood. Insert the tip of pipette to the bottom of Wintrobe tube and fill it from bottom by gradually withdrawing the pipette upwards keeping the tip under the rising column of blood.
4. Fill the Wintrobe tube till 0 cm mark.
5. Transfer the tube to the Wintrobe stand.
6. Let it stand in strictly vertical position for 1 hour at room temperature.
7. After one hour note the reading, i.e. the level to which red cell column has fallen.

Observation

After one hour red cells will settle down below the column of plasma. Note the reading on tube corresponding to the upper limit of the red cell sediment. This will give the value of ESR.

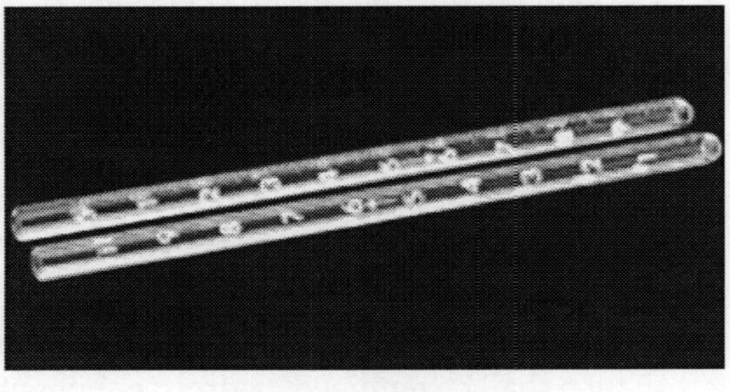

Fig. D2.3: Wintrobe tubes

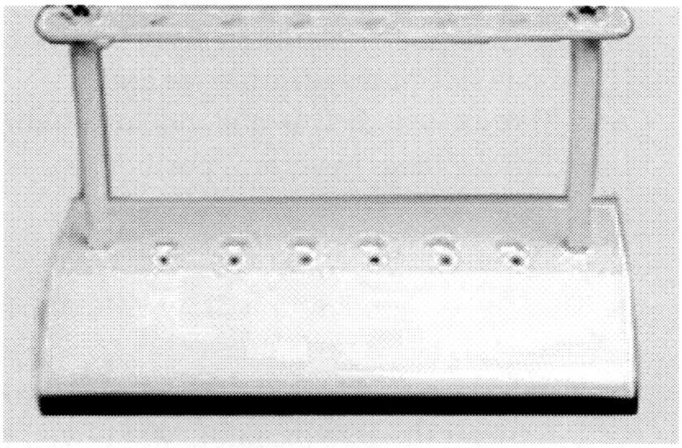

Fig. D2.4: Wintrobe stand

Result

The distance of fall of erythrocytes, expressed as millimeters in 1st hour.

ESR is expressed as .... mm/hr

Normal Value by Wintrobe Method is:

Males: 0-9 mm at the end of 1st hour

Females: 0-20 mm at the end of 1st hour

Precautions

1. Fasting sample should be taken.
2. Tube should be clean and dry.
3. Do not use hemolyzed specimen it will give false low reading.
4. While filling the Wintrobe tube to avoid air bubble formation and damage to red cells, the pasteur pipette should be withdrawn gradually keeping its tip under the rising column of blood.
5. There should be no air bubble in the tube and if present discard that sample.
6. Wintrobe tube should not be filled from the top as blood will not flow down to its bottom because of air present in the tube.
7. Excess amount of blood if present in the tube shall be removed by dropper not with any absorbent material. Proper amount of anticoagulant should be used and mixed properly with blood. If higher concentration of anticoagulant is added it will give false low value.
8. Sample should be stored no longer than 2 hours at room temperature or 6 hours at 4°C.
9. There should be no air bubble in the tube and it should be filled up to zero mark.
10. Tube should be kept vertical and undisturbed for 1 hour.
11. Test should be done at room temperature.
12. Reading should be taken after 1 hour not earlier (It should not be taken after 30 minutes and result multiplied by 2) because sedimentation is complete only after 1 hour.

Advantages of Wintrobe Method

Same sample can be used for ESR first and then for Hct.

Disadvantages

Wintrobe tube is only 100 mm long. The shorter column makes this method less sensitive than the Westergren method because the maximal possible abnormal value is lower. However, this method is more practical for demonstration purposes.

Sources of Error

1. Improper anticoagulant.
2. Tilting of tube. Inclination by 30 raises ESR by 30%.
3. Dirty tubes.
4. Vigorous mixing of blood sample with anticoagulant leading to bubble formation.
5. Hemolyzed blood sample.
6. Test performed after 2 hours of sample collection.

OTHER METHODS

The desire for alternate methods is driven primarily by 2 characteristics of the standard methods:

1. Long analytical time (60 minutes sedimentation time plus setup and reading time).
2. Requirement for relatively large specimen volumes (1.0-2.0 ml).
3. The need for diluting specimens and the elevation of the ESR by anemia.

Zeta Sedimentation Ratio (ZSR)

A centrifugal device (Zetafuge) spins capillary tubes filled with blood in a vertical position. In four 45-second cycles it accelerates the formation of rouleaux and RBC sedimentation. The capillary tube is then read as a microhematocrit, giving a value called the zetacrit. The true hematocrit is divided by zetacrit, and the result is the ZSR.

Advantages of ZSR Method

1. The ZSR method can be completed in a few minutes.
2. It requires only 100 µl of blood.
3. It is not affected by anemia and correlates reasonably well with the Westergren method when the ESR is only mildly or moderately elevated.

Disadvantages of ZSR Method

It requires special equipment which is no longer produced.

VES-matic ESR

The VES-matic family of systems contains several modifications of the Westergren method. One ml of whole blood is collected into a special tube containing enough sodium citrate to both anticoagulate and dilute the blood in the 4:1 modified Westergren ratio. The tube is placed on a reader where it is held at an angle of 18° off vertical to accelerate sedimentation. An infrared reader determines the endpoint after 20 minutes. The VES-matic ESR results correlate well with the modified Westergren results and offer advantages of improved timeliness and less specimen handling. Drawbacks include the need for specialized equipment and specimen tubes.

Micro-ESR

The basis of the micro-ESR method is the reduction of the required specimen volume by using a column with an internal diameter of only 1 mm rather than the 2.5 mm or more of a standard method. One micro-ESR method uses a column 230 mm long while another uses a 75 mm column. Both methods are targeted for pediatric use, where a reduction in specimen volumes is highly desirable.

DISCUSSION

Stages of ESR

Stage 1: It lasts for 1-10 minutes. It is a period of aggregation. Rouleaux formation occurs in this stage. Sedimentation is slow.

Stage 2: It occurs during next 40-45 minutes. During this period sedimentation rate is fast

Stage 3: It is during last 10 minutes. There occurs final packing of RBCs at the bottom.

Erythrocytes Sedimentation is Controlled by two Types of Factors

Opposing Factors

1. RBCs repel each other due to the negative charges on their surfaces called zeta potential.
2. The large surface-area-to-volume ratio of normal RBCs resists settling.
3. An upward force due to viscosity of plasma.

Favouring Factors

1. Rouleaux formation: The aggregation of RBCs into rouleaux, which happens slowly under normal conditions accelerates sedimentation.
2. A down ward gravitational force acting on red cells due to their weight favors sedimentation.

FACTORS THAT PLAY ROLE IN ESR

Plasma Factors

1. Fibrinogen: Fibrinogen's positive charge decreases the RBCs' zeta potential, leading to increased rouleaux and an increased ESR. In fact, the clinical utility of the ESR is largely attributable to increased fibrinogen in acute-phase reactions and chronic inflammatory conditions.
2. Globulin: It also favors ESR.
3. Cholesterol increases ESR.
4. Acute phase proteins, products of tissue inflammation and destruction neutralizes zeta potential to increase ESR.
5. Increase in plasma viscosity decreases ESR.
6. Albumin retards ESR.
7. Lecithin retards ESR.

Red Cell Factors

Count

1. Anemia favors ESR by creating more space between RBCs, anemia reduces the effect of the zeta potential to slow sedimentation.
2. Polycythemia resists ESR by decreasing the compactness of rouleaux formation.

Shape and size-sedimentation rate is directly proportional to the weight of the cell aggregate and inversely proportional to the surface area.

1. Macrocytosis: Increases ESR.
2. Microcytes: Decreases ESR.
3. Spherocytosis, sickle cell disease, marked variation in RBC size (anisocytosis) hinders rouleaux formation so decreases ESR.
4. Thalassemias and hemoglobinopathies. The surface-area-to-volume ratio is increased so ESR is decreased.

Increase in ESR is seen in conditions that decrease the zeta potential or the RBC surface-area-to volume ratio. The zeta potential is reduced by other plasma proteins, including immunoglobulins, as well as cholesterol, phospholipids, and some medications.

PHYSIOLOGICAL CONDITIONS

1. High temperature due to change in plasma viscosity.
2. Females due to lower Hct.
3. Pregnancy – ESR rises after first trimester.
4. Menstruation.
5. Advanced age.

PATHOLOGICAL CONDITIONS

1. Extreme obesity.
2. Anemias.
3. Acute bacterial infections.
4. Chronic infections – pneumonia, tuberculosis, Syphilis etc.
5. Collagen vascular diseases, e.g. Systemic Lupus Erythmatosis, Rheumatoid Arthritis.
6. Gout.
7. Malignancy – Hodgkin's disease, gastric carcinoma, renal cell carcinoma, chronic lymphocytic leukemia, breast cancer, colorectal cancer and prostate cancer.
8. Multiple myeloma.
9. Myocardial infarction.
10. Rheumatic fever.
11. Temporal arteritis.
12. Acute heavy metal poisoning.
13. End-stage renal failure.

14. After use of drugs like:
    - Dextran
    - Heparin
    - Penicillamine
    - Procainamide
    - Theophylline
    - Vitamin A.

Decrease in ESR is seen in the conditions that interfere with the formation of rouleaux or increase the RBC surface-area-to-volume ratio.

Physiological Conditions

1. Hypothermia.
2. Cachexia.
3. Recent feeding.
4. Newborn.
5. Males.

Pathological Conditions

1. Congestive heart failure.
2. Afibrogenemia.
3. Sickle cell anemia.
4. Spherocytosis.
5. Thalassemia.
6. Allergies.
7. Achlouric jaundice.
8. After use of drugs like:
    - Valproic acid
    - Steroids
    - Anti-inflammatory agents
    - Corticotropin
    - Cortisone
    - Ethambutol
    - Quinine
    - Salicylates.

Clinical Significance of ESR

The ESR is one of the oldest and simplest laboratory tests still in common use. Its clinical value is derived primarily from its elevation by increased concentrations of fibrinogen and immunoglobulins, but the utility is limited by its clinical non specificity and it is being affected by a large number of technical and physiological variables. As a nonspecific test, the ESR has inherent limitations in its clinical utility; however, in some clinical contexts the ESR may provide valuable information for diagnosis, and monitoring disease activity or therapeutic response.

DIAGNOSTIC USE OF ESR

1. Temporal arteritis and giant cell arteritis – A giant cell arteritis involving the temporal arteries, is a medical emergency. Unless treatment is instituted within a few hours, there is a high risk of ophthalmic arterial thrombosis, leading to blindness. The definitive diagnosis is made by histological examination of a temporal artery biopsy, but this examination cannot generally be performed quickly enough to guide initial therapy. In patients with temporal arteritis, the average ESR is > 90 mm in Ist hour (Westergren method) and exceeds 30 mm in Ist hour in 99%. When symptoms of temporal arteritis are present, an elevated ESR particularly a highly elevated ESR indicates that corticosteroid therapy should be started immediately.
2. The ESR is used in the emergency department setting in the evaluation of suspected appendicitis, pelvic inflammatory disease, septic arthritis, and other inflammatory diseases.
3. For monitoring diseases – The ESR continues to be used as an aid in monitoring the activity of selected inflammatory diseases. The ESR is usually highly elevated in these patients. A significant decrease in the ESR, in combination with improved clinical

Red Cell Factors	*Increases ESR*	*Decreases ESR*
Red blood cell count	Anemia	• Polycythemia
Red blood cell size and shape	Macrocytosis Erythroid aggregates	• Microcytosis • Spherocytosis Acanthocytosis • Anisocytosis (marked) • Sickle cells • Spherocytosis • Thalassemia
Bile salts		high concentration (affects RBC membranes)
White blood cell count	Leukemia	Leukocytosis (marked)
Plasma Factors		
Fibrinogen	hyperfibrinogenemia	Hypofibrinogenemia Dysfibrinogenemia
Globulin	Hypergammaglobulinemia	Hypogammaglobulinemia
Albumin	Hypoalbuminemia	Hyperalbuminemia
Cholesterol and phospholipids	Hypercholestremia	Increased phospholipids
Coagulation system	Heparin	DIC (low fibrinogen)
Technical Factors		
Tube handling	Tilted ESR tube Vibration High room temperature	Narrow ESR column diameter Bubbles in ESR column Low room temperature
Anticoagulant	Heparin as anticoagulant	Clotted specimen
Testing and specimen handling	Refrigerated sample not returned to room temperature	Delay in testing

status, is indicative of a therapeutic response. Sustained elevation of the ESR, even with symptomatic improvement, suggests a poor response to therapy. ESR is used in monitoring:

1. Temporal Arteritis and Polymyalgia Rheumatica.
2. Rheumatoid Arthritis.
3. Other collagen vascular diseases.
4. Neoplastic Diseases.

A high ESR has been found to correlate with an overall poor prognosis for various types of cancers.

WORK SPACE

ANSWER THESE QUESTIONS

Q1. What is ESR?

Q2. What is the principle of determining ESR?

Q3. What are the methods for determining ESR?

Q4. Which method is better and why?

Q5. What precautions are taken for determining ESR?

Q6. Why ESR reading should be taken after 1 hour not earlier?

Q7. What is the advantage and disadvantage of Westergren method of determining ESR?

Q8. What is the advantage and disadvantage of Wintrobe method of determining ESR?

Q9. What are the factors affecting ESR?

Q10. What is the clinical significance of ESR determination?

Q11. What are the conditions in which ESR is increased?

Q12. What are the conditions in which ESR is decreased?

CHAPTER

14

Determination of Osmotic Fragility of RBCs

DEMONSTRATION-3

OBJECTIVE

Students should know:

- Different test for determination of osmotic fragility
- Different precautions observed
- Clinical significance of osmotic fragility.

Introduction

The normal red blood cell is a relatively impermeable biconcave disc which maintains osmotic equilibrium with the surrounding medium. As the surrounding medium becomes hypotonic, fluid will be taken into the cell to maintain stability. Eventually under very hypotonic conditions the cell will fill to capacity and rupture.

Methods

Red cell osmotic fragility can be evaluated by means of different methods:

1. By using decreasing concentrations of NaCl.
2. Acidified glycerol lysis test (AGLT).
3. The pink test.
4. Nestroft (naked eye single tube red cell osmotic fragility test).

Osmotic Fragility Test by Using Decreasing Concentrations of NaCl

Principle

Heparinized blood is placed in a series of tubes of decreasing concentrations of sodium chloride solutions and incubated at room temperature for one hour. Hemolysis is used as an index of the degree of susceptibility of erythrocytes to hypotonic damage.

Apparatus

1. Heparin.
2. Material for collection of venous blood.
3. Test tube stand with 12 test tubes.
4. Dropper.
5. Distilled water.
6. 1% NaCl.

Procedure

1. In a test tube stand take 12 clean and dry test tubes.
2. With the same dropper prepare decreasing concentration of saline solution by putting varying number of drops of saline and distilled water according to the table given below.

Test tube no.	1	2	3	4	5	6	7	8	9	10	11	12
No. of drops of distilled water	3	9	10	11	12	13	14	15	16	17	18	25
No. of drops of 1% NaCl	22	16	15	14	13	12	11	10	9	8	7	0
Concentration of NaCl obtained in %	0.88	0.64	0.60	0.56	0.52	0.48	0.44	0.40	0.36	0.32	0.28	0

3. Place your thumb over each test tube and mix the contents by gentle inversion.
4. Under aseptic conditions draw 2 ml of venous blood.
5. Gently transfer it to a heparin containing vial.
6. Put one drop of blood to each test tube.
7. Mix the blood and saline solution by placing your thumb over the top of the test tube and inverting it few times.
8. Allow the tubes to stand at room temperature for one hour.
9. After one hour, observe the test tubes against white back ground.

Precautions

1. Heparinized blood or defibrinated blood is preferred for osmotic fragility test because of the absence of "salts". EDTA, oxalates or sodium citrate will increase the "salt" concentration of blood and possibly skew the results.
2. The osmotic fragility test should be conducted as soon as possible after collecting the blood specimen. It is recommended that testing should be done within two hours after collection. If the test cannot be performed within this time frame, the blood should be refrigerated.
3. Osmotic fragility testing can be adversely affected by temperature and pH.
4. Hemolyzed sample should not be used.
5. Same dropper should be used for adding distilled water and 1% saline to prepare different concentration of saline solutions.
6. Saline solution and blood should be mixed by gently inverting test tubes.
7. Vigorous shaking of test tubes should be prevented else it will cause mechanical lysis of RBCs.
8. Readings should be taken after one hour.
9. Readings should be taken by holding test tubes against the white background.

Observations

Osmotic fragility is determined by measuring the degree of hemolysis in hypotonic saline solution. Observe the RBCs at the bottom and the supernatant saline in each of the test tubes.

Initial (beginning of) Hemolysis: There will be RBCs in the bottom of the tube and the fluid will be tinged red.

Complete (total) Hemolysis: There will be no RBCs in the bottom of the tube. The fluid will be a transparent red.

Result

Note the tube number and % NaCl in which hemolysis has begun.

Note the tube number and % NaCl in which complete haemolysis is seen.

Express your result as

Beginning of osmotic fragility .... % NaCl

Completion of osmotic fragility .... % NaCl

Normal Value

Osmotic fragility begins at 0.45-0.50% of NaCl
Osmotic fragility is complete at 0.30-0.33% of NaCl

The Acidified Glycerol Lysis Test (AGLT)

AGLT is based on the measure of the time taken by the erythrocytes to lyse when exposed to glycerol. After the suspension of the blood sample in a buffered isotonic solution and the addition of glycerol, the kinetic of hemolysis is recorded as the decrease of absorbance at 620 nm. The results are expressed as GLT50, i.e. the time necessary to have 50% hemolysis that corresponds to the time taken for the absorbance to fall to half of its original value. Spherocytes, being unable to resist swelling, lyse in a shorter time than erythrocytes.

Advantages of this Method

The test can be performed on blood stored for up to 24 hours.

It has higher sensitivity,

It requires lesser amount of blood and shorter execution time.

For these reasons it is particularly useful as a screening procedure for the diagnosis of hereditary spherocytosis in large family studies and population surveys.

The Pink Test

It is a further modification of the acidified glycerol test. It is an end-point method based on the measure of the hemolysis of a small volume of blood in a buffered solution contained 135 mmol/L glycerol.

Advantages of this Method

The Test shows a diagnostic sensitivity similar to AGLT. It is very easy to perform and the results do not critically depend on the pH of the lysis solution, unlike obtained with AGLT.

NESTROFT (Naked Eye Single Tube Red Cell Osmotic Fragility Test)

The single tube test is based on the use of a single hypotonic solution having a critical saline concentration able to differentiate between normal and thalassemic subjects. The test is interpreted by visualization, negative samples being clear and positive cloudy. It is a simple, rapid, low cost and reliable test for thalassemia mass screening, particularly useful in developing countries where the prevalence of thalassemic disorders is high and the resources limited.

DISCUSSION

Normal erythrocyte is characterized by a biconcave shape giving it an excess of surface area in relationship to its volume. The osmotic fragility test evaluates the relationship of the RBCs surface area to its volume. When there is a decrease in the surface area to the cell volume (as in the spherocyte), the osmotic fragility is increased. The resistance of such cells to hypotonic solutions is decreased. In cells, as the target cell, where the surface area relationship to the volume of the cell is increased over that typified in the normal erythrocyte, there is an increased resistance to hypotonic solutions. Such cells have a decreased osmotic fragility.

Significance of Osmotic Fragility Tests

Osmotic fragility tests are based on the measure of red blood cell lysis as a function of osmotic stress. They are mainly useful in:

1. The diagnosis of hereditary spherocytosis
2. They are also used as a screening test for beta-thalassemia in under-resourced countries where automated blood-cell counters are available in only a limited number of major centres

Red cell osmotic fragility is considered to be increased if hemolysis occurs in a sodium chloride concentration > 0.5%. Osmotic fragility is considered to be decreased if hemolysis is not complete in a 0.30% NaCl solution.

Increased Osmotic Fragility is Characteristically Associated with

1. Hereditary spherocytosis – Because of their reduced surface membrane area respect to the cell volume, spherocytes cannot expand as much as normal discoid erythrocytes and result osmotically more fragile.
2. Hemolytic anemias associated with the presence of spherocytes. particularly autoimmune hemolytic anemia.
3. Hypernatremia (Na > 155 meq/L).

Decreased Osmotic Fragility is Associated with

1. Thalassemia, in both the homozygous and heterozygous forms,
2. Iron deficiency
3. Hyponatremia (Na < 130 meq/L),
4. Polycythemia vera
5. Sickle cell anemia after splenectomy.

WORKSPACE

ANSWER THESE QUESTIONS

Q1. What is osmotic fragility?
Q2. What are the different tests for determination of osmotic fragility?
Q3. What is the significance of determining osmotic fragility?
Q4. What precautions are taken for osmotic fragility test?
Q5. Why blood should not be vigorously mixed with saline solution?
Q6. What are the conditions where osmotic fragility is increased?
Q7. What are the conditions where osmotic fragility is decreased?

CHAPTER

15

Normal Hematological Values

Total Red Blood Cell count

In males: 4.75 - 6.0 millions/mm^3 of blood
In females: 4 - 5.5 millions/mm^3 of blood

Total White Blood Cell Count

Adults: 4000 - 11,000/cu mm
Children: 5000 -15,000/cu mm
Infants: 6000 - 18,000/cu mm
Newborns: 10000 - 25, 000/cu mm

Differential Leukocyte Count

Neutrophil: 50 - 70%
Eosinophil: 1 - 4%
Basophil: 0 - 1%
Monocyte: 2 - 8%
Lymphocyte: 20 - 40%

Hemoglobin Concentration

Males: 14 - 18 g/dl
Females: 12- 16 g/dl
New borns: 16 - 22 gm/dl

Bleeding Time

Duke's method: 1 - 5 minutes
Ivy's method: 3 - 8 minutes.
Simplate method: < 7 minutes

Clotting Time

Capillary glass tube method: 2 - 8 minutes.
Lee and White tube method: 5 - 12 minutes

Packed cell volume

Males: 47·7%
Females: 42·5%
Full term baby/newborn: 54·10%
Infants: 38·6%
Children: 41·4%

Blood Indices

Mean Corpuscular Volume: 78-96 fl (femtoliters)
Mean Corpuscular Hemoglobin: 27-33 pg (picograms)
Mean Corpuscular Hemoglobin Concentration: 30-37%

Erythrocyte Sedimentation Rate

Westergren Method

Males: 3-5 mm at the end of 1st hour
Females: 5-12 mm at the end of 1st hour

Wintrobe Method

Males: 0-9 mm at the end of 1st hour
Females: 0-20 mm at the end of 1st hour

Osmotic Fragility

Osmotic fragility begins at 0.45-0.50% of NaCl
Osmotic fragility is complete at 0.30-0.33% of NaCl.

Bibliography

1. Barer R. Lecture Notes on The Use of the Microscope. Blackwell Scientific Publications,Oxford 1959
2. Dacie JV, Lewis SM. Practical Haematology (8th Ed). Churchill Livingstone, Edinburgh 1996
3. Mary Louise Turgeon. Clinical Hematology Theory and Procedures (4th Ed). Lippincott Williams & Wilkins 2004.
4. Procedure for the Collection of Diagnostic Blood Specimens by Venipuncture, Approved Standard (5th Ed) 2003; H3-A5.
5. Procedure for Collection of Diagnostic Blood Specimens by Skin Puncture, Approved Standards (3rd Ed) 1991;11: H4-A3.
6. Procedure for Collection of Diagnostic Blood Specimens by Venipuncture, Approved Standards (3rd Ed) 1991;11: H4-A3,
7. Procedures and Devices for the Collection of Diagnostic Capillary Blood Specimens, Approved Standard (5th Ed) 2004;H4-A5.
8. Ranade VG, Pradhan P, Joshi PN. A Text Book of Practical Physiology (3rd Ed). Pune Vidyarthi Griha Prakashan
9. Samson Wright, Cyril A Keele. Applied Physiology (12th Ed). Oxford Medicine.
10. Viroj Wiwanitkit. A note in the acid citrate dextrose tube in the present usage. Haema 2003;6(3):407-08.

Index